SOMATIC EXERCISES
TO LOSE WEIGHT

Techniques to remove mental barriers, regain balance and confidence

&

LOSE WEIGHT.

9-DAY PROGRAM INCLUDED

Maia Solara

Index

Part 1

Part 2

Part 3

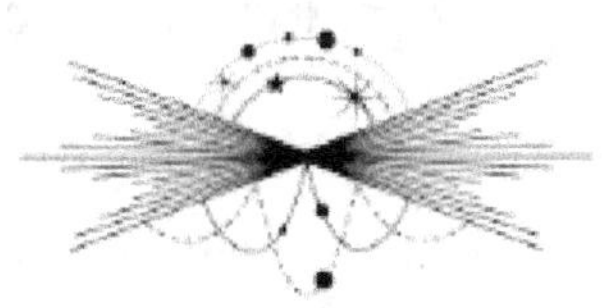

Introduction

Welcome to this extraordinary journey toward physical and mental transformation. If you are reading these lines, chances are you are looking for an effective and sustainable way to lose weight, feel better, and live a healthier life. This book was written to guide you step by step through a unique approach that combines a balanced diet with somatic yoga practices and emotional healing.

My goal is to offer you a holistic path that not only helps you lose body fat but also completely transforms your well-being. Here you will discover how to exercise and mentally lose weight, how to avoid common dietary mistakes, and how to eliminate bad habits.

'Mental and emotional well-being plays a crucial role in your physical transformation.'

If you have already read other books in this series, you should have learned a lot about somatic yoga. It is important to keep the body map in mind whenever you practice somatic yoga, because the focus during the exercises must be on what you feel, on what the exercise moves you as sensations, thoughts and emotions. You have to let go of these sensations, release tension, let new energy flow and clean the energy channels.

Get ready to unlock your potential and discover a new version of yourself, leaner, stronger and at peace with your body and mind.

Unlocking Trauma and Mental Blocks

To achieve lasting transformation and meaningful transformation, it is essential to address not only the physical aspects of weight loss, but also the mental and emotional aspects. Often, past traumas and mental blocks can hinder our progress, creating stress, anxiety and a cycle of unhealthy eating habits.

Somatic yoga is a powerful practice that focuses on body awareness and releasing accumulated tension. This form of yoga helps you become more aware of your body's signals, promoting a deeper connection with your physical and mental needs. Through slow, deep movements, you can release stress and negative emotions, creating a positive mental environment that supports weight loss.

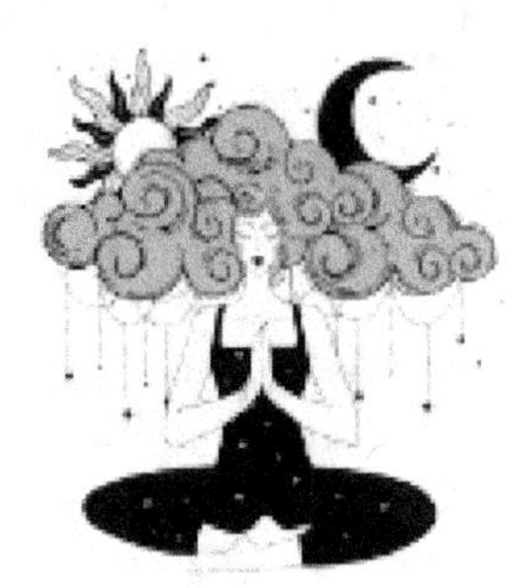

The process of inner healing is essential for breaking the cycle of trauma and mental blocks, enabling you to embrace a new life of well-being and vitality. Somatic yoga not only improves your flexibility and strength, but also guides you toward greater awareness and inner peace, facilitating your physical transformation.

Bad habits to change

To properly approach somatic practice to lose weight, it is crucial to recognize and correct some common wrong ways of thinking. I will list some of these common habits; if you recognize yourself in some of them, it is important that you adopt the given suggestions to overcome them and turn over a new leaf for good.

How to put balanced goals?

The first mistake that is often made is to focus exclusively on rapid weight loss. This can push people to make drastic and unhealthy choices, risking compromising overall well-being. Instead, it is crucial to take a balanced and sustainable approach, and put realistic goals in place, such as a balanced diet and a gradual increase in physical activity. This not only promotes healthier and more lasting weight loss, but also ensures long-term maintenance of the weight achieved, thereby improving overall health and well-being.

Have you ever wondered how you could improve your weight loss journey by taking a more balanced approach? Reflect on this and try to give yourself an answer as to how you might incorporate healthy and sustainable habits into your daily routine. Reflecting and planning, before you act, is very important because it allows you to make choices that suit your personal situation.

How to overcome procrastination?

Many people make the mistake of not being consistent in their weight loss journey. Frequently jumping from strict dieting to overeating or playing too much sport can undermine progress and reduce motivation in the long run. Skipping workouts and postponing the start of new diet regimen is very common custom among people who fail to lose weight.

To maintain consistency, it is helpful to reward yourself for each small success. For example, set realistic weekly goals and reward yourself with a little attention when they are achieved. This not only reinforces the desired behavior, but also keeps motivation high in the long run, making success in achieving one's weight goals more likely.

Here are five possible rewards that can be used to reinforce small successes in the weight loss journey:

Time for yourself: Spend time on a hobby or activity you love, such as reading a book, taking a relaxing walk or watching a movie.

Small personal shopping: Buy something nice and reasonable, such as a new book, a household item, or an item of clothing.

Beauty treatment: Treat yourself to a beauty treatment, such as a manicure, pedicure or relaxing facial mask.

Different physical activity: Try a new activity, such as a tango class or walking a new route.

Time with friends: Arrange to meet with friends or family members to spend pleasant time together. Make a phone call to a friend.

These rewards not only recognize the work done toward weight loss goals, but are also a pleasant way to enjoy each day to the fullest.

How might you make your weight loss journey more consistent and motivating? Think about ways to incorporate small rewards into your routine to make it more enjoyable and sustainable.

Having a negative self-image and having negative thoughts crowding your mind can be a significant obstacle in the path to weight loss and overall well-being. These thoughts can undermine motivation and lead to feelings of defeat.

It happens to everyone to have those days when you feel down about your body or person. It is important to recognize that these negative thoughts can profoundly affect our well-being. For example, you may find yourself constantly comparing yourself to others, thinking that you are not good looking or fit enough like them. These kinds of thoughts can make you feel inferior and dissatisfied.

Then there are those times when we focus on specific parts of our body that we don't like. Maybe it's the weight, shape, or size of certain areas that we just can't accept. Constantly criticizing ourselves for these aspects can really undermine our self-esteem.

Finally, we sometimes have catastrophic thoughts, worrying excessively about negative consequences related to our physical appearance. We fear being judged by others or not being accepted because of our appearance. These thoughts can become really debilitating.

The key to dealing with these thoughts is to **be aware of when** they occur and **replace them with positive motivational phrases**.

Repeating to yourself that you are enough, that you are doing your best, and that every step toward your well-being is important can make a big difference. Here are some phrases that can help:

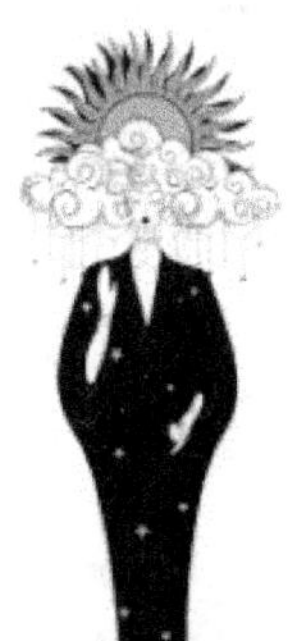

"I am strong and capable of achieving my goals."

"Every small step I take brings me closer to the best version of me."

"I deserve love and respect, exactly as I am."

"My value does not depend on my physical appearance."

"I accept and appreciate my body for everything it does for me every day."

Using these phrases regularly can help strengthen motivation, develop a more positive outlook, and keep the focus on the path of self-improvement

Remember that the path to a positive self-image is made up of small steps and lots of self-love.

Choose a place and time of day when you can safely repeat these phrases out loud so that they support your day. You can also write them on your bathroom mirror or in your cell phone cover for easy access and not to forget to repeat them several times a day.

Dieting also plays a crucial role in weight loss, but it is important to understand that it does not have to be a restrictive and unsustainable diet. Many of us fall into the traps of drastic diets that promise quick results but often lead to frustration and long-term failure.

What is caloric deficit?

Many "experts" suggest that losing weight depends only on the type of food you consume, but the truth is that to lose weight, you need to be in a calorie deficit. If you consume more calories than you burn, you will gain weight. Conversely, if you consume fewer calories than you burn, you will lose weight. Numerous studies show the importance of calorie balance.

A prime example is the experiment of Mark Haub, professor of human nutrition at Kansas State University, who lost 27 pounds in two months by eating only foods such as Twinkies and Doritos while maintaining a calorie deficit of 800 calories per day. This shows that being in a calorie deficit is critical for weight loss. Of course, this was just an experiment that under no circumstances should be replicated. It is essential to follow a healthy and balanced diet.

Do you ever find yourself eating snacks after a meal, chips for appetizers, or ice cream after dinner? These are precisely the times when you absent-mindedly add calories to your day.

Think about how you could easily eliminate or replace these habits with an herbal tea, a fruit or a cup of coffee. What could you change in your daily routine to avoid these extra calories?

It may seem like a good idea, even based on the above, to drastically cut calories to lose weight fast, but I assure you that it is not the right way to go. When you cut calories too much, your body goes into survival mode, thinking it is about to face a famine. As a result, it slows down your metabolism to conserve energy, making it much harder to lose weight and much easier to regain it once you return to normal eating.

Instead, it is much more effective to eat according to a personalized calorie goal that takes into account your specific needs and goals. This allows you to lose weight in a healthy and sustainable way without putting your metabolism at risk. Remember, the key is to find a balance and make food choices that support your long-term well-being.

How many times have you skipped a meal thinking about losing weight? There are diets such as the intermittent fasting diet, which if used consciously can make the goal of weight loss achieved, otherwise, skipping meals haphazardly can only create metabolic imbalances.

If you belong to this category, it is important to carefully decide which diet to choose and no longer suffer by skipping meals.

Are all calories the same?

Although calories are important, they are not the only thing that matters. When it comes to fat loss, it is also crucial to consider macronutrients (protein, carbohydrates, and fat). For example, consuming too many carbohydrates can make it difficult to lose fat because they increase insulin, a hormone that blocks fat loss and promotes energy storage in the form of body fat. Optimizing macronutrient intake is crucial for effective fat loss.

It is really important to know the foods you consume and understand how they affect your body. In this regard, I have produced a booklet that can be a first step in deepening your knowledge about foods. You can download it for free by using the QR code on the following pages.

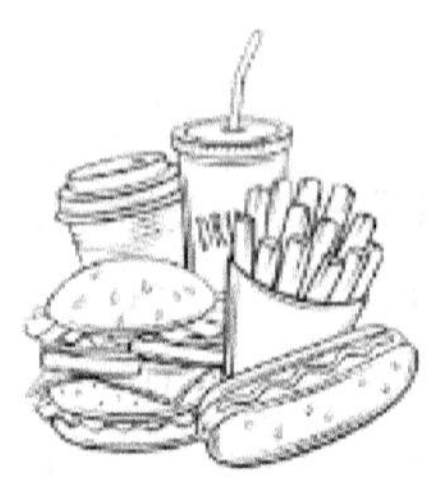

Which diet to choose?

Very restrictive diets deplete willpower, increase cravings and lead to binge eating, sabotaging one's weight loss efforts. Most people who follow overly restrictive diets fail because they cannot maintain them in the long term. To achieve long-term success, you need to follow a practical, simple and sustainable approach that allows you to enjoy your favorite foods. The key is to find a balance that allows you to transform your body without giving up the pleasure of food.

Avoiding these common dietary mistakes will help you optimize hormone levels, increase metabolism, and lose fat safely and effectively. Following a balanced diet that accounts for calories and macronutrients, and is sustainable over the long term, is critical to success in your weight loss.

How could you improve your weight loss journey by taking a more balanced approach? Reflect on this and try to give an answer on how you could incorporate healthy and sustainable habits into your daily routine.

As we have said, it is important to keep fit and lose the extra pounds if necessary so that you look good, feel healthier, and develop a sense of pride and self-esteem. Once the ideal weight is reached, it will also be necessary to maintain the weight achieved.

Most people accumulate those extra pounds by eating the wrong things. Changing these bad eating habits is the key to long-term success.

Since cave times, human beings have developed a natural system for storing energy in the form of fat, ensuring their survival in times of food shortages. This mechanism, inherited from our ancestors, is still present today, although we no longer live in a hunting and gathering context. Our bodies continue to store fat, and the number of fat cells we possess is partly determined by genetics. However, despite the difficulties associated with genetic predisposition and the accumulation of new fat cells, we are not doomed to remain overweight.

To achieve effective weight control, it is necessary to act on several fronts: physical, mental and, most importantly, dietary. Changing the type of food we consume is essential to ingest less fat and, at the same time, provide our bodies with the nutrients they need to function properly. In fact, some natural foods not only promote weight loss, but also help maintain it in the long term.

Therefore, I have created a manual for you that is intended to be a guide on how to choose the right foods to promote fat melting and offers an example of a balanced diet to achieve and maintain your wellness goal.

As a thank you for your trust, I have prepared this BONUS for you to download and use every day.

1-Week Mediterranean Diet & The Foods That Burn Fat

Journal Progress Diary

Audio of the Book and Guided Breathing Videos

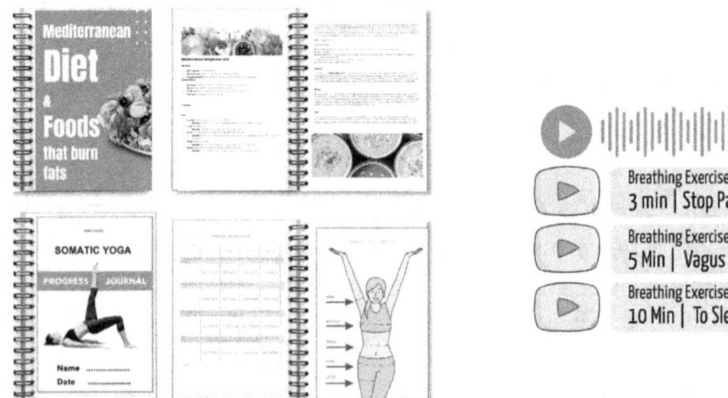

https://ngcompany.aweb.page/p/73589184-218e-4be2-bd41-78d8462483ef

Click the link to access your bonus materials!

Part 2

Somatic practice and mindfulness

Somatic therapy is a therapeutic approach that recognizes the connection between mind and body, aiming to treat the obstacles of our mind through bodily sensations and experiences.

For this reason, it is important that before you begin the exercises, you brush up on some knowledge that is fundamental to success in this course. This information is explained more d etly in other books in this collection and taught with practical exercises. If you have not yet had a chance to view the other books and do the exercises, you should know that the basis is the proper use of body maps. Through these maps you can identify the critical points where you have pain, where you are most stiff, contracted, and where you have accumulated the most fat (waistline, thighs, back, arms).

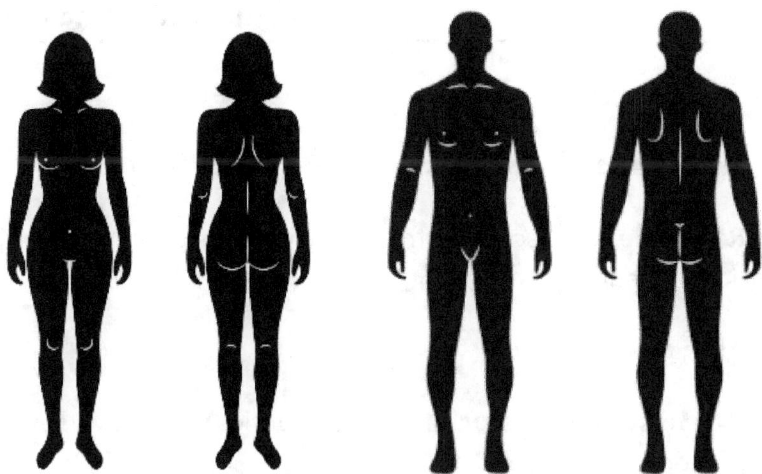

Fat storage is due to genetic structure but can also have psychosomatic explanations. The way our bodies store fat may reflect our emotional and psychological states.

For example, fat accumulated in the abdominal area is often associated with chronic stress and anxiety, as the stress hormone, cortisol, promotes the accumulation of visceral fat. Fat around the hips and thighs may indicate insecurities related to sexuality and emotional support. Fat accumulated in the upper body, such as arms and shoulders, may reflect a need for protection or a feeling of being overwhelmed by responsibility. The legs and buttocks, if they are the areas of accumulation, may indicate rooting problems or feelings of lack of stability in life.

These accumulations are not only the result of excessive caloric intake, but can be deeply influenced by our emotions and stress, highlighting how important an integrated approach that considers both physical and emotional health is for effective weight management.

Fat accumulation and causes

Abdominal area:

- **Psychosomatic Association**: Chronic stress and anxiety.

- **Rationale**: Cortisol, the stress hormone, promotes visceral fat accumulation.

Hips and Thighs:

- **Psychosomatic Association**: Insecurities related to sexuality and emotional support.

- **Rationale**: Fat in these areas may indicate a need for protection or emotional comfort.

Upper Body (Arms and Shoulders):

- **Psychosomatic Association**: Need for protection or feeling of being overwhelmed by responsibility.

- **Rationale**: Accumulation in these areas may reflect a defense mechanism against excessive stress.

Legs and Glutes:

- **Psychosomatic Association**: Rootedness problems or feelings of lack of stability in life.

- **Rationale**: Fat in these areas may represent the search for stability and security.

General Influences:

- **Not Only Calorie Intake**: Fat accumulation is not only due to excess calories.

- **Emotions and Stress**: Emotions and stress play a significant role in how the body stores fat.

- **Integrated Approach**: Considering both physical and emotional health is essential for effective management of weight.

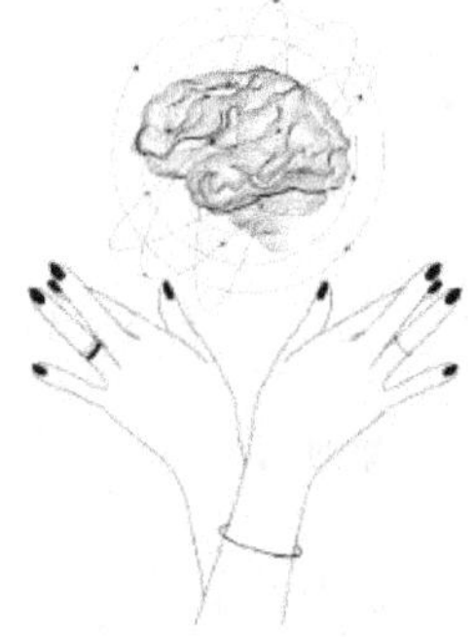

Find a quiet place: Choose a place where you will not be disturbed and feel comfortable.

Get comfortable: Sit or lie down in a position that allows you to relax completely.

Comfortable clothing: Make sure your clothes are comfortable. If the waistband is too tight or the elastic in your underwear is bothering you, loosen or remove what is causing you discomfort. Check that you are neither too hot nor too cold.

Eliminate distractions: Turn off your cell phone or put it on silent mode to avoid electronic interruptions.

Observe the body map: Use a body map illustrated in the book or draw one on a sheet of paper. Alternatively, use a full-length photo of yourself and imagine that you see yourself in that image.

Describe body sensations: For each body part on the map or photo, use adjectives to describe the sensation you feel. For example, for the neck, it could be: cold, stiff, sore, hot, tense, swollen. Use this list of possible body sensations and enrich it with words you prefer:

Tense	Bloated	Heavy
Relaxed	Rigid	Numb
Cold	Painful	Tingling
Hot	Lightweight	Contract

Free	Locked	Sensitive
Vibrant	Smooth	Anesthetized
Button	Rough	

Continue throughout the body: Proceed systematically from head to toe, describing the sensations in each part of the body.

Close your eyes: When you feel ready, close your eyes to better focus on the sensations in your body. Repeat the exercise with your eyes closed.

Breathe deeply: Inhale slowly through the nose and exhale slowly through the mouth. Repeat a few times, letting the descriptions of the sensations come effortlessly.

Bring attention to the feet: Notice how your feet feel. Are they relaxed or tense? Warm or cold? Do you feel contact with the floor?

Shift your attention upward: After the feet, move to the ankles, calves, knees, and so on, up to the head. Notice the sensations in each part of the body without trying to change them.

Consciously relax each body part: As you bring attention to each area, try to consciously relax it, letting go of any tension.

Notice the breath: Bring your attention to the natural rhythm of the breath without trying to change it.

Stay in the present moment: Continue to breathe consciously and maintain attention on the sensations of the body and breath for a few minutes.

Finish the exercise slowly: When you feel ready, start moving your fingers and toes slowly. Open your eyes gradually and take a few moments to return to awareness of your surroundings.

Reflect on the experience: Take a moment to reflect on how you feel, noting any changes in the level of tension or body awareness.

Becoming aware of the areas of your body that you want to reshape and where you want to lose weight is essential for an effective and sustainable approach. Understanding why and how you have accumulated fat allows you to address not only the physical aspects, but also the emotional and psychological aspects that can affect your weight. This process of awareness will help you identify and address the root causes, thereby improving your overall health and well-being.

5 Questions to Reflect on Your Pathway

1. What are the areas on your body where you have noticed fat accumulation?

   Reflecting on this will help you focus on the specific areas to be reshaped.

2. When did you start to notice fat accumulation in these areas?

   Identifying when it started can help you link the change to specific events or periods of stress in your life.

3. What stressful emotions or situations have you experienced that may have contributed to fat accumulation?

   Understanding the link between emotions and weight can be crucial in addressing psychological causes.

4. How do you generally react to stress?

   Your responses to stress, such as compulsive eating or having sedentary behaviors, can influence fat accumulation.

5. What changes can you make in your daily routine to improve your physical and emotional health?

Thinking about small practical changes, such as adopting stress management techniques, improving nutrition or increasing physical activity, can make a big difference in your weight loss journey.

Becoming aware of your habits and behavior patterns is the first step in making positive changes. A mindful, integrated approach will help you reshape your body in a sustainable way and improve your overall well-being.

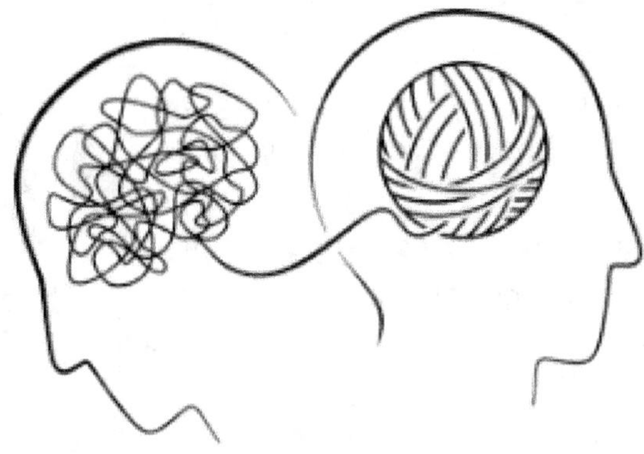

Part 3
Somatic practice to lose weight

To get the most benefit from your practice, it is important to create the ideal environment and conditions. Here are some basic elements to get you started:

A Quiet Place: Find a quiet space where you will not be disturbed. This will allow you to concentrate fully on your practice and enter a state of deep relaxation. Make sure the space is well ventilated and large enough to allow you to move freely.

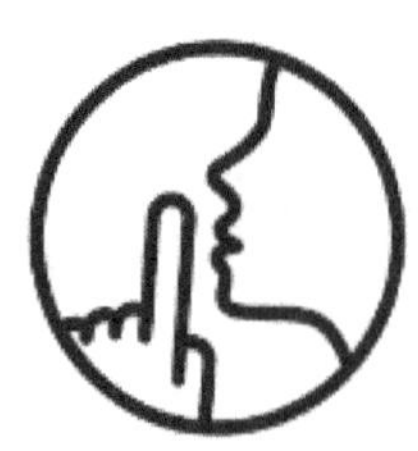

Comfortable Clothing: Wear comfortable clothing that allows freedom of movement. Ideal clothing for somatic yoga is soft, stretchy and breathable. Avoid tight or stiff clothing that may restrict your movement or cause discomfort.

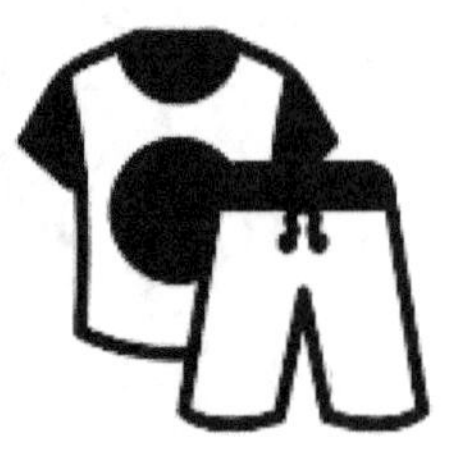

A Yoga Mat: A non-slip yoga mat provides adequate cushioning for joints and provides a stable surface on which to practice. If possible, choose a mat that is easy to clean and transport. If you do not have a mat, you can still practice on a mat or towel.

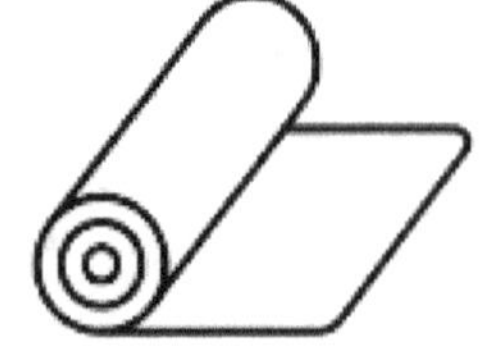

Support Accessories: Although not strictly necessary, some accessories can make the practice more comfortable. Pillows, yoga blocks and blankets can be used to support the body in different positions, improving alignment and reducing stress on specific areas.

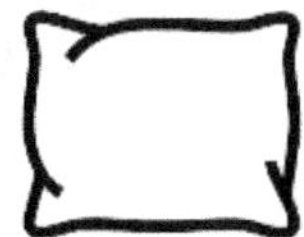

An Open and Receptive Attitude: Perhaps the most important element of all is an open and receptive attitude. Approach the practice with curiosity and without judgment, allowing yourself to explore movement and body awareness in a gentle and compassionate way.

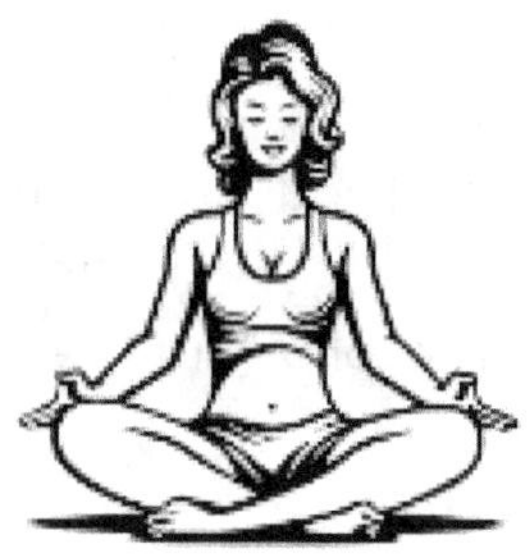

Preparing these elements before you begin will help you create a more rewarding and beneficial somatic yoga experience.

Good practice!

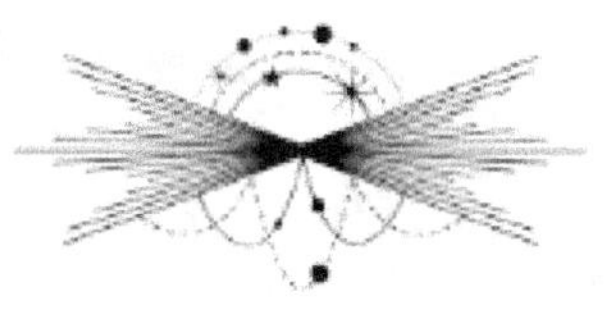

Losing weight is not just about sweating and struggling in a gym. Above all, losing weight is about reconnecting with your original fitness and finding the balance that suits you.

Exercise 1

Sit on the floor with your legs flexed against your chest.

Exhale and grasp your knees with your hands. (Figure 1)

Inhale and open your chest. Bring your arms behind your back (Figure 2)

Perform the exercise by placing your attention on your back muscles as they contract and lengthen. Feel the abdominals working. Perform the movement slowly following the breath. Let the tension in your back slowly release.

Repeat slowly for 15 times

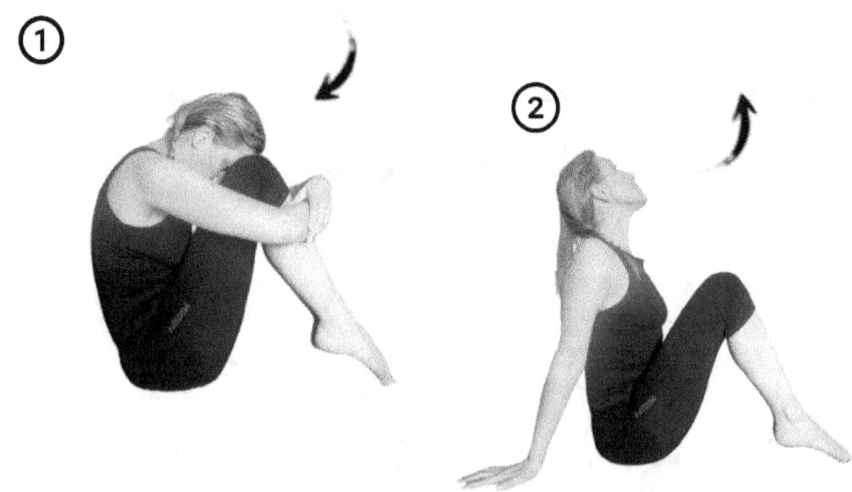

Sit on the floor with your legs flexed against your chest and your hands resting on the floor near your feet. (Figure 1)

Exhale and extend the right leg in front of you. (Figure 2)

Inhale and return to the starting position. (Figure 3)

Perform the exercise with attention on the hamstrings stretching and the abdominals contracting. Try to feel old tensions giving way to renewed flexibility. If you feel the tense leg vibrate, it means you are releasing old tensions.

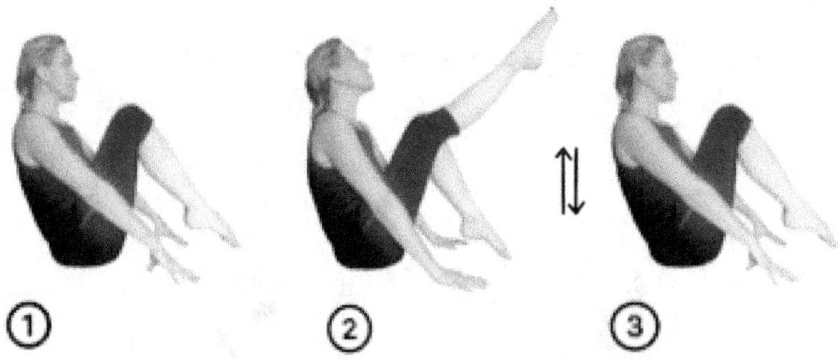

Lift to lower right leg quickly 15 times

Lift to lower for 15 times the left leg

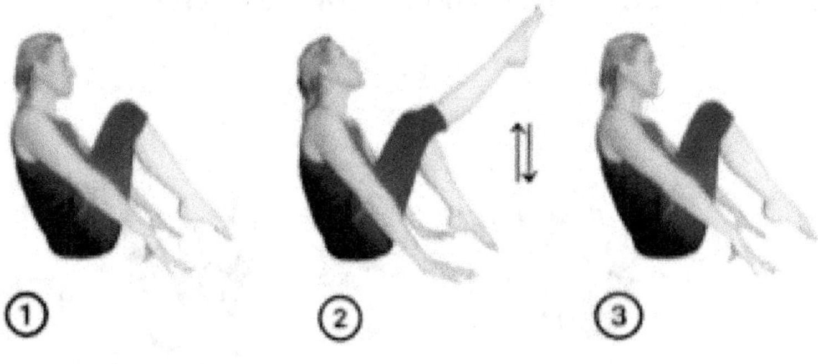

Sit on the floor with your legs flexed against your chest and your hands resting on the floor near your feet. Take long breaths focusing on stretching in the spine. Imagine air flowing through the entire spine, loosening knots and tension. (Figure 1)

Slowly extend the right leg in front of you and take long breaths. (Figure 2)

Perform the exercise with your attention on the hamstrings stretching and the abdominals contracting. If your outstretched leg trembles, it means you have reached the point of maximum tension beyond which you cannot yet go. Your flexibility and strength will increase day by day; don't rush it.

Hold the position for 15 seconds with the right leg

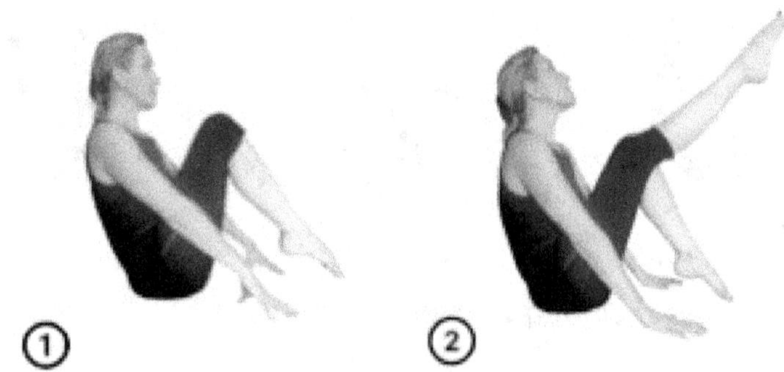

Hold the position for 15 seconds with the left leg

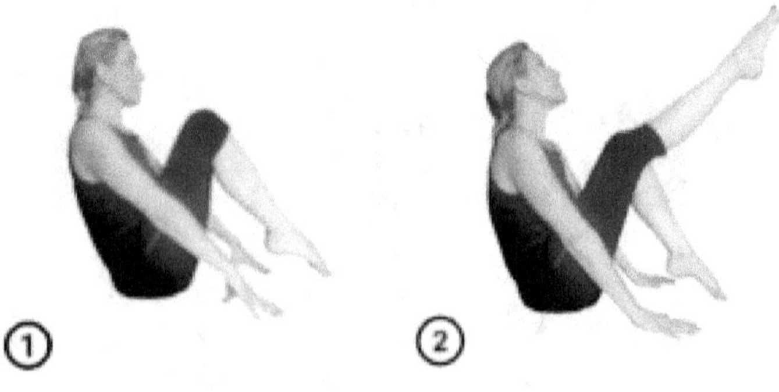

Sit on the floor with your legs flexed against your chest and your hands resting on the floor near your feet. (Figure 1)

Exhale and extend both legs in front of you. (Figure 2)

Inhale and return to the starting position. (Figure 3)

Perform the exercise by listening to the muscles warming up and accepting the fatigue. Visualize fat being burned and muscles firming.

Perform the movement 15 times x 3 times

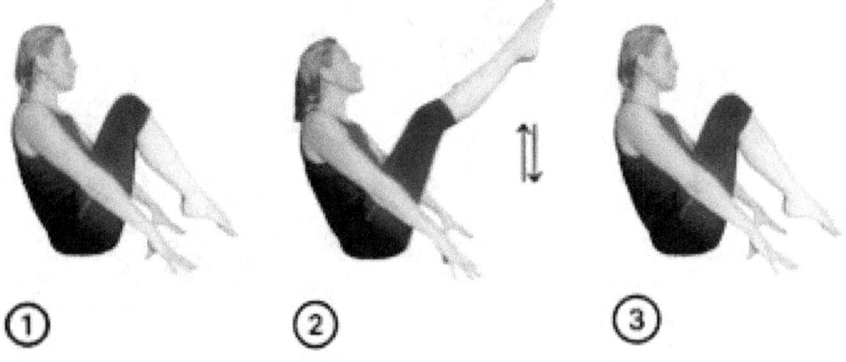

Then hold the position for as long as possible.

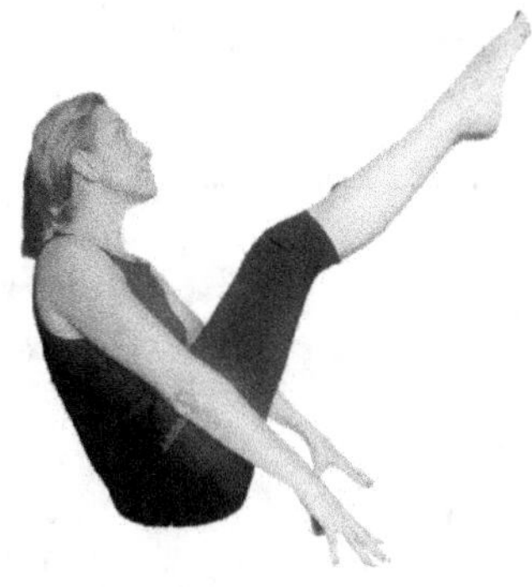

Lie comfortably on your back, with your arms resting at your sides and your eyes closed. (Figure 1)

Take a few deep breaths to center yourself and relax your body. Listen to the effects the practice has had on your body and mind. (Figure 2)

Remain in this position a few minutes.

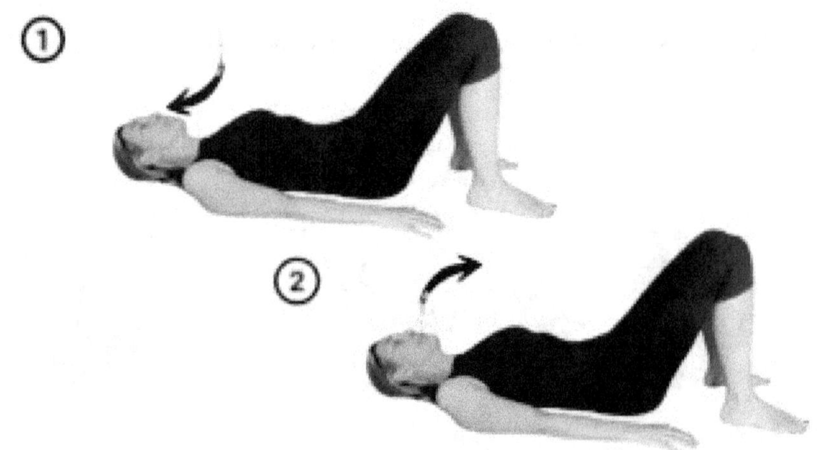

Phrase of the Day

To be repeated several times throughout the day:

"The secret to moving forward is to begin." - Mark Twain

Gratification

Enjoy a nice warm bath.

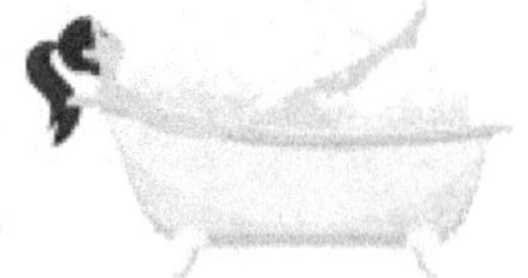

Ingredients:

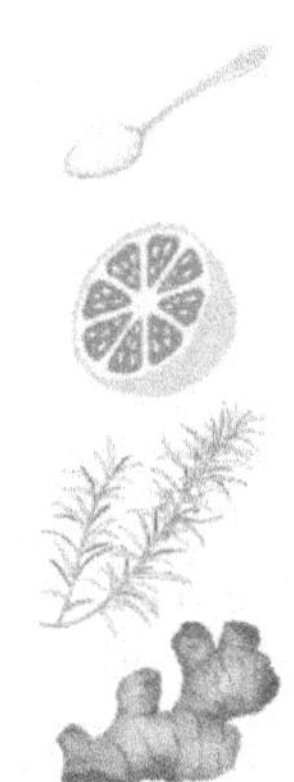

- 1 cup of salt
- 1 cup of baking soda
- 10 drops of grapefruit essential oil
- 10 drops of rosemary essential oil
- 10 drops of ginger essential oil
- 1 tablespoon ginger powder (optional)
- Hot water

Preparation of the Bath:

- Fill the bathtub with hot, but not boiling, water to avoid discomfort and make sure it is at a comfortable temperature for you.

Addition of Salt and Sodium Bicarbonate:

- Add 1 cup of salt and 1 cup of baking soda to the water. These help relax muscles, improve circulation and reduce swelling.

Essential Oils:

- Add 10 drops of grapefruit essential oil, 10 drops of rosemary essential oil, and 10 drops of ginger essential oil. These essential oils are known for their stimulating properties and can help improve metabolism and promote detoxification.

Addition of Ginger Powder (Optional):

- For an additional warming and detoxifying effect, you can add 1 tablespoon of powdered ginger. Stir the water well to evenly distribute the ingredients.

Diving:

- Enter the tub and soak completely. Soak for at least 20 to 30 minutes to allow your body to absorb the benefits of the ingredients.

Relaxation:

- During the bath, try to relax completely. You can listen to relaxing music, meditate or simply close your eyes and enjoy the moment.

Hydration:

- After bathing, dry yourself gently with a soft towel and apply moisturizer to keep your skin soft.

Benefits:

- **Muscle Relaxation:** Salt helps relax muscles and reduce tension.

- **Detoxification:** Baking soda and essential oils promote detoxification of the body.

- **Improved Circulation:** Grapefruit, rosemary and ginger essential oils stimulate blood circulation and metabolism.

- **Stress Reduction:** A hot bath is a great way to reduce stress and improve overall well-being, which is essential for an effective mindset in weight loss.

Taking a hot slimming bath regularly can be a pleasant and beneficial part of your weight loss routine, helping to improve physical and mental health.

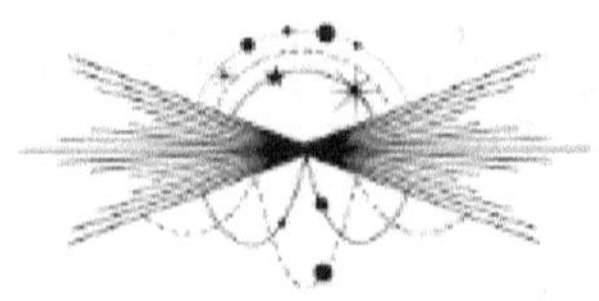

Position yourself in quadrupedal position. Exhale and round your back upward, like a stretching cat. Push your hands and knees against the floor to increase the curve of your back. Bring the chin toward the chest, trying to look at the navel. Imagine the space being created between the vertebrae. (Figure 1)

Inhale deeply as you arch your back downward. Look slightly upward or forward, without forcing the neck. Keep your shoulders away from your ears and open, creating space in your chest. Listen to the air coming in through your nose and regenerating you. Let everything that has hurt you in life move away from you, like soap bubbles. (Figure 2)

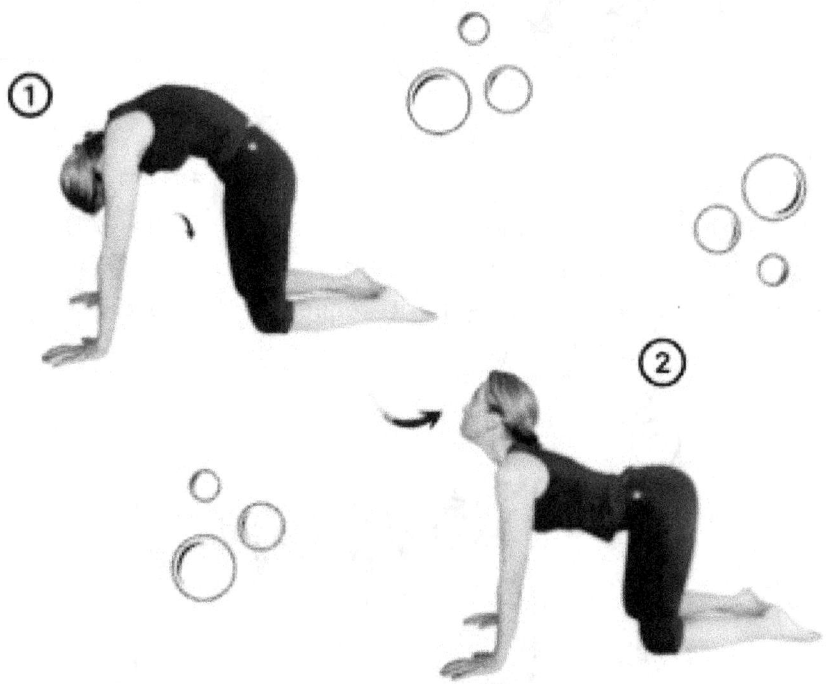

Continue alternating the position for 15 times

Position yourself sitting on the floor, with your hands behind your back and knees slightly open. Your feet are firmly on the ground. (Figure 1)

Inhale and rise into the half-bridge position, lifting the pelvis off the ground. Tense looking at the navel. (Figure 2)

Perform the movement 15 times x 3 times

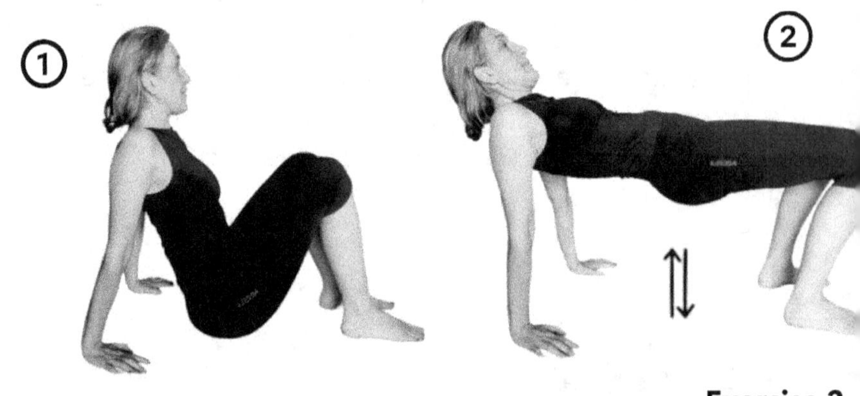

Exercise 3

Position yourself in the mid-bridge and take long, deep breaths. Feel your glutes contract and your abdominals tense. Listen to the strength in your arms and legs and reflect on the solidity of your ground supports. (Figure 3)

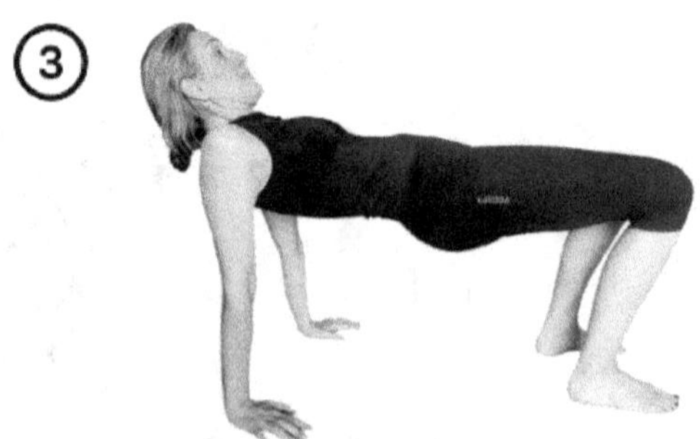

Hold the position as long as possible

Perform the movement 15 times x 3 times

Position yourself sitting on the floor, with your hands resting on the floor near your thighs and your legs stretched forward. (Figure 1)

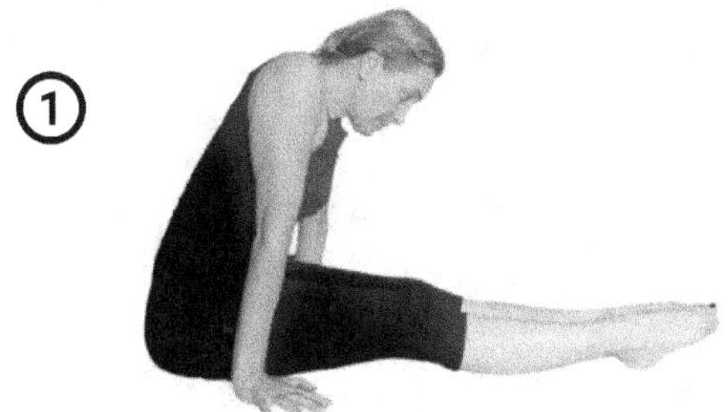

Inhale and bend your knees. Push the pelvis toward the feet and keep the pelvis lifted off the ground. Listen to the tension in your shoulders and stretch your head upward. (Figure 2)

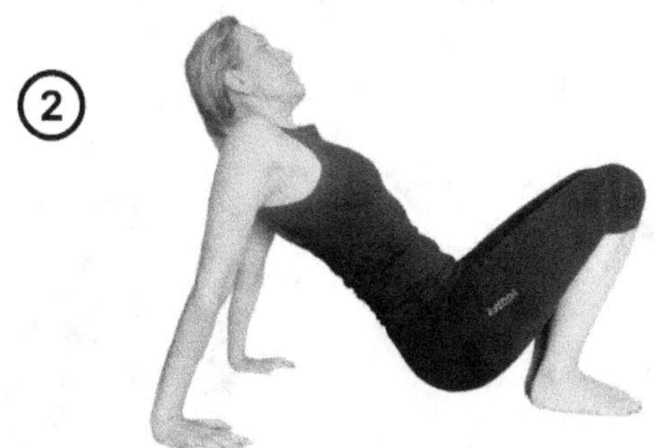

Exhale and return with hands resting on the floor near the thighs and legs stretched forward. (Figure 3)

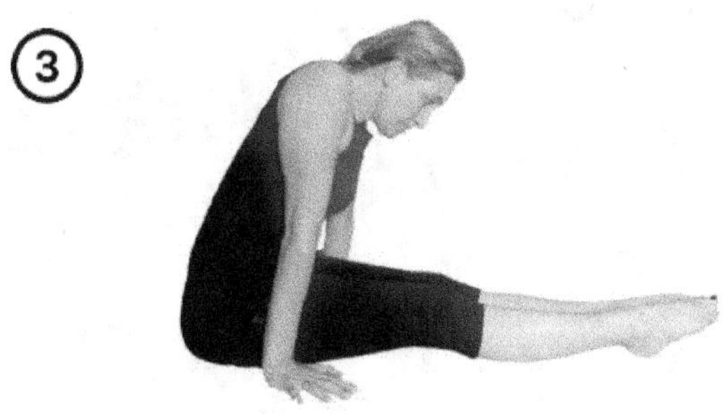

Position yourself sitting on the floor, with your hands resting on the floor near your thighs and your legs stretched forward. (Figure 1)

Go into the half-bridge position, past the positions shown in Figures 2, 3, 4 and 5. Perform the movement fluidly, breathing deeply and listening to all the muscles and joints moving smoothly together. Imagine that you are fluid and light.

Perform the clockwise rotary motion 15 times

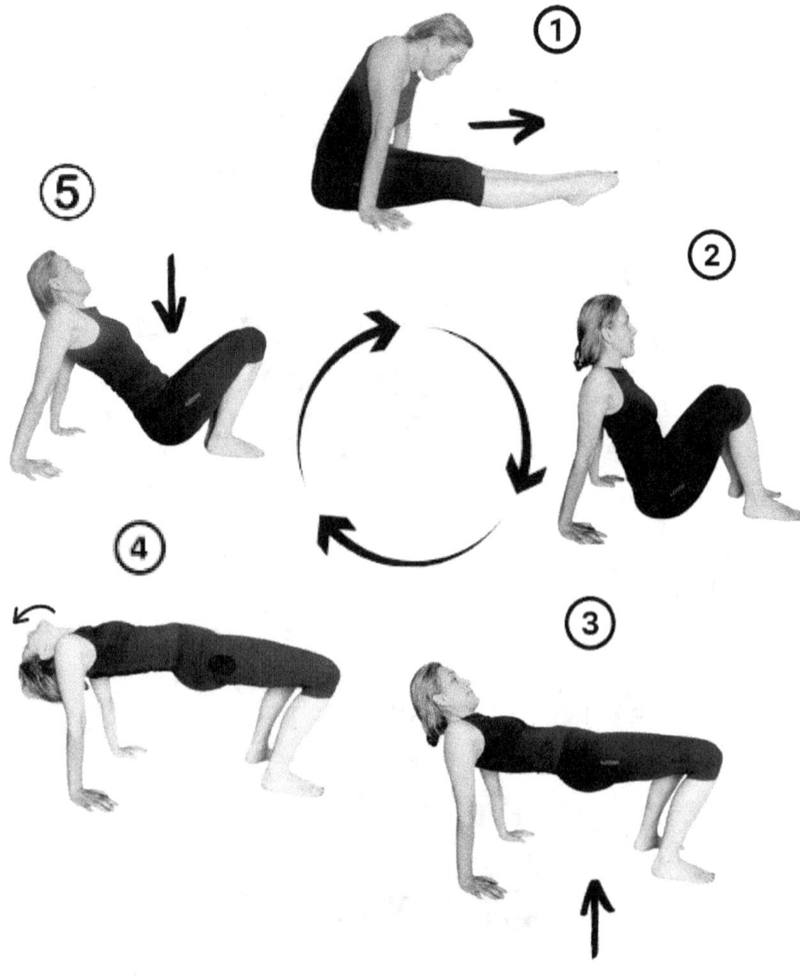

Go into the half-bridge position, leaving the head facing downward, if you want to increase the intensity of the movement. (Figure 1)

Go into the sitting position, past the positions shown in Figures 2, 3, 4 and 5. Perform the movement fluidly, breathing deeply and listening to all the muscles and joints moving smoothly together. Imagine that you are fluid and light.

Repeat the counterclockwise rotary motion 15 times

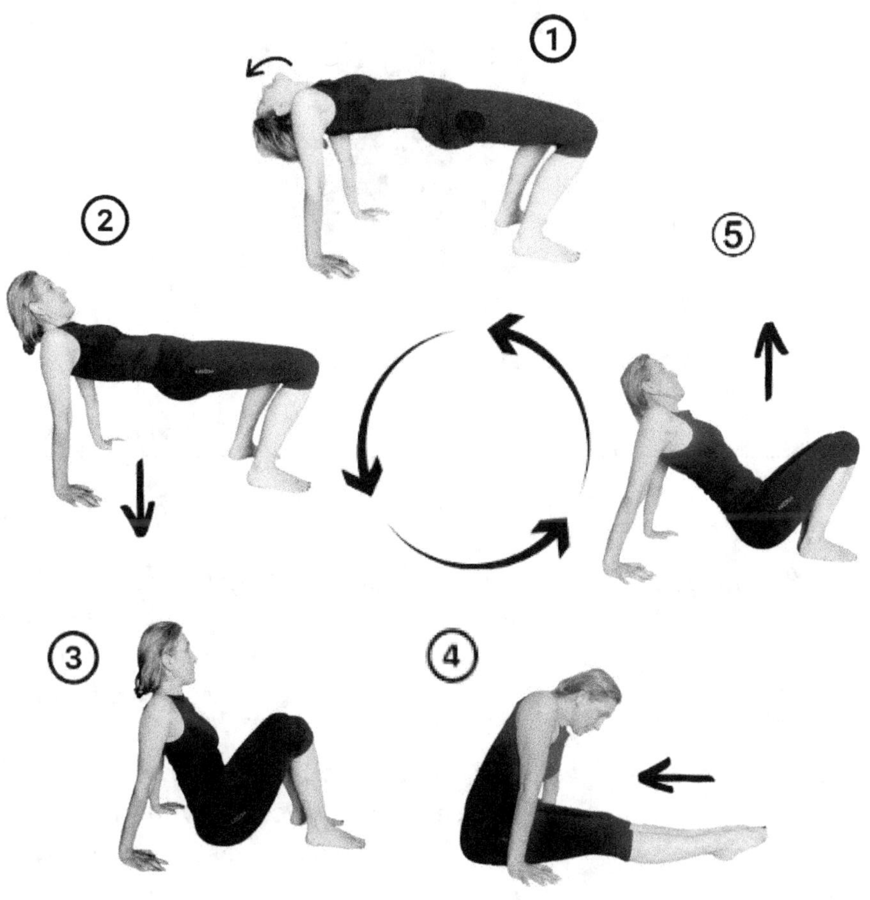

Sit comfortably with your spine erect, cross-legged on the floor. Place your hands on your knees and close your eyes. (Figure 1)

Breathe slowly. Imagine that you have large wings so that you can fly lightly.

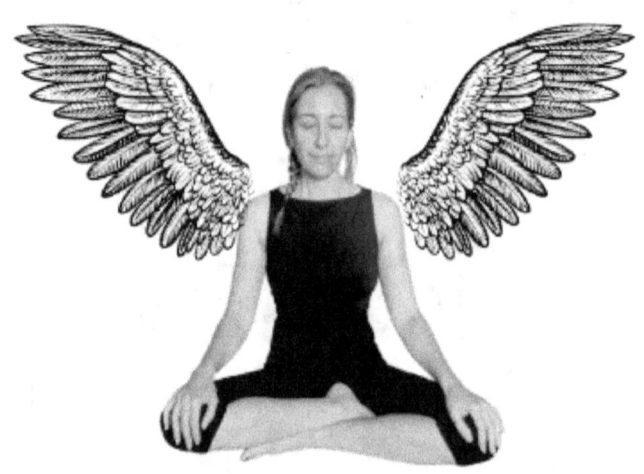

Remain in this position a few minutes

Phrase of the Day

To be repeated several times throughout the day:

"It's not about perfection. It's about improving yourself." - Jillian Michaels

Gratification

Gather a bouquet of flowers or buy a seedling, to beautify your home and enjoy the scents of flowers.

Do not neglect the power of flowers.

Aromatherapy uses essential oils extracted from plants and flowers to promote physical and mental well-being. When it comes to weight-loss diets, aromatherapy can be a useful adjunct, helping to manage appetite, reduce stress, and improve mood. These effects can help maintain motivation and make the weight loss journey more enjoyable and sustainable.

Flowers and Essential Oils to Use:

Lavender:

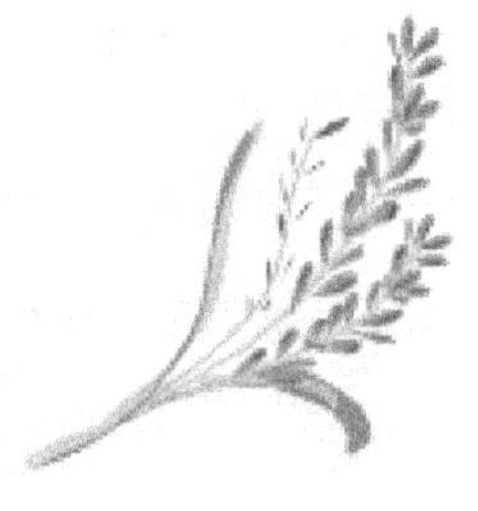

> **Benefits:** Reduces stress and anxiety, promotes relaxation and improves sleep quality. Good sleep is essential for hunger hormone regulation and weight management.

> **Usage:** Aromatherapy diffuser, relaxing bath, or topical application (diluted with carrier oil).

Grapefruit flowers:

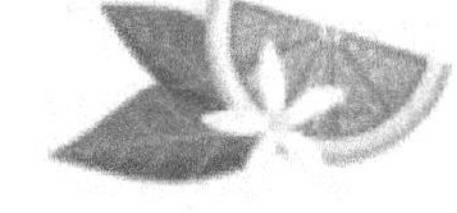

> **Benefits:** Stimulate metabolism, reduce appetite and increase energy levels. Grapefruit essential oil is known for its cleansing and detoxifying properties.

> **Usage:** Aromatherapy diffuser, massage (diluted with carrier oil), or direct inhalation.

Peppermint Flower:

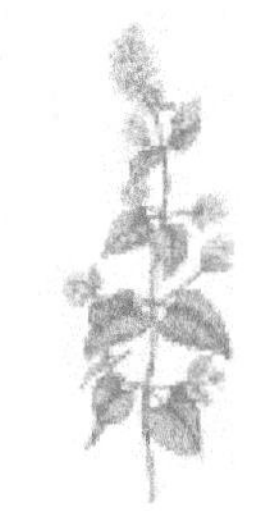

> **Benefits:** Reduces hunger and cravings, improves concentration and energy levels. It can also relieve digestive discomfort, which is often common during diets.

Usage: Aromatherapy diffuser, direct inhalation, or topical application (diluted with carrier oil).

Rosemary Flower:

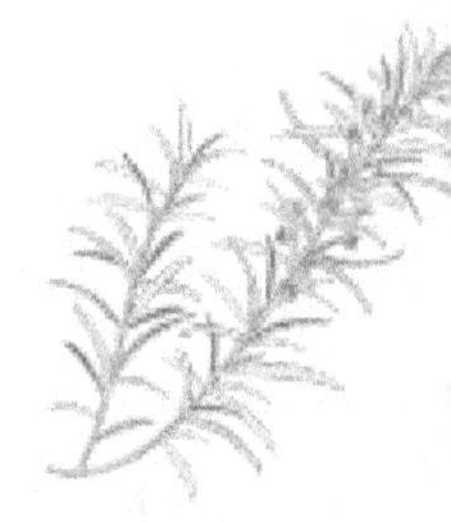

Benefits: Improves memory and concentration, increases energy and aids digestion. It can also help reduce stress.

Usage: Aromatherapy diffuser, massage (diluted with carrier oil), or direct inhalation.

Jasmine:

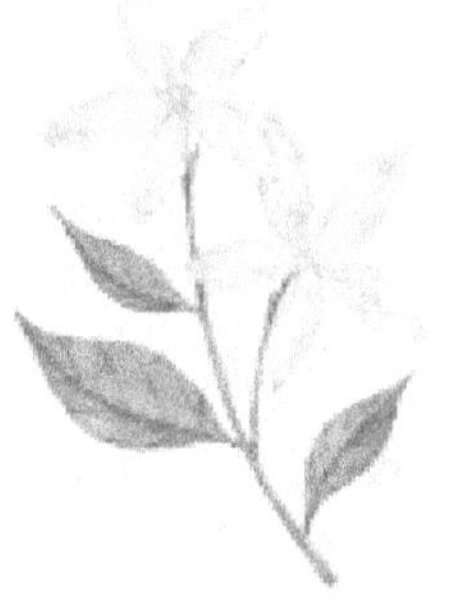

Benefits: Elevates mood, reduces stress and boosts self-confidence. Emotional well-being is critical to maintaining a healthy, balanced diet.

Usage: Aromatherapy diffuser, topical application (diluted with carrier oil), or direct inhalation.

Chamomile:

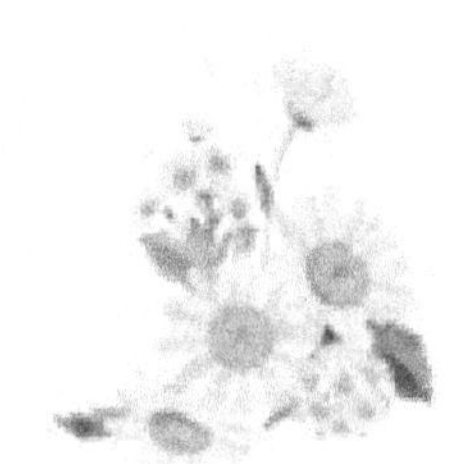

Benefits: Promotes relaxation, improves sleep and reduces anxiety. It is especially useful for those who tend to stress eat.

Usage: Aromatherapy diffuser, relaxing bath, or topical application (diluted with carrier oil).

How to Use Essential Oils:

- **Diffuser:** Add a few drops of essential oil to the diffuser to fill the room with the beneficial scent.

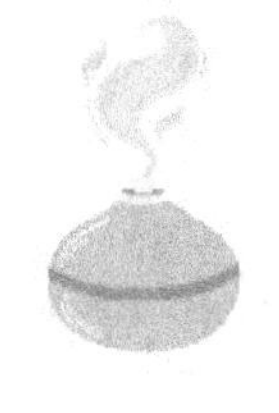

- **Massage:** Dilute essential oils in a carrier oil (such as coconut or almond oil) and massage the body to absorb the beneficial properties through the skin.

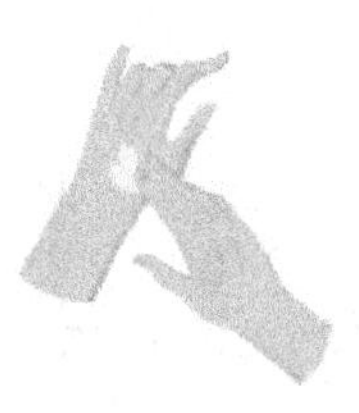

- **Aromatic Bath:** Add a few drops of essential oil to the bath water for a relaxing and therapeutic experience.

- Inhalation: Inhale essential oils directly by applying a few drops to a handkerchief or using a personal vaporizer.

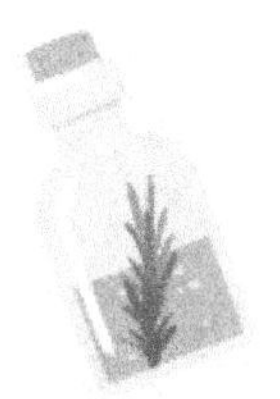

Aromatherapy can be a powerful and enjoyable component of a weight loss program, helping to balance mind and body on the journey to healthier living.

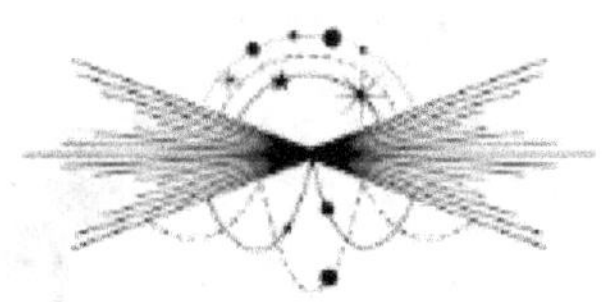

Position yourself with your back on the floor, arms stretched along your sides and knees bent. (Figure 1)

Inhale and lift the pelvis upward. (Figure 2)

Return to position 1. (Figure 3) Perform the movement slowly, listening as the vertebrae come off the ground one at a time. We often live in tension and some vertebrae experience crushing. Mentally clear the space between vertebrae and make room for clean energy.

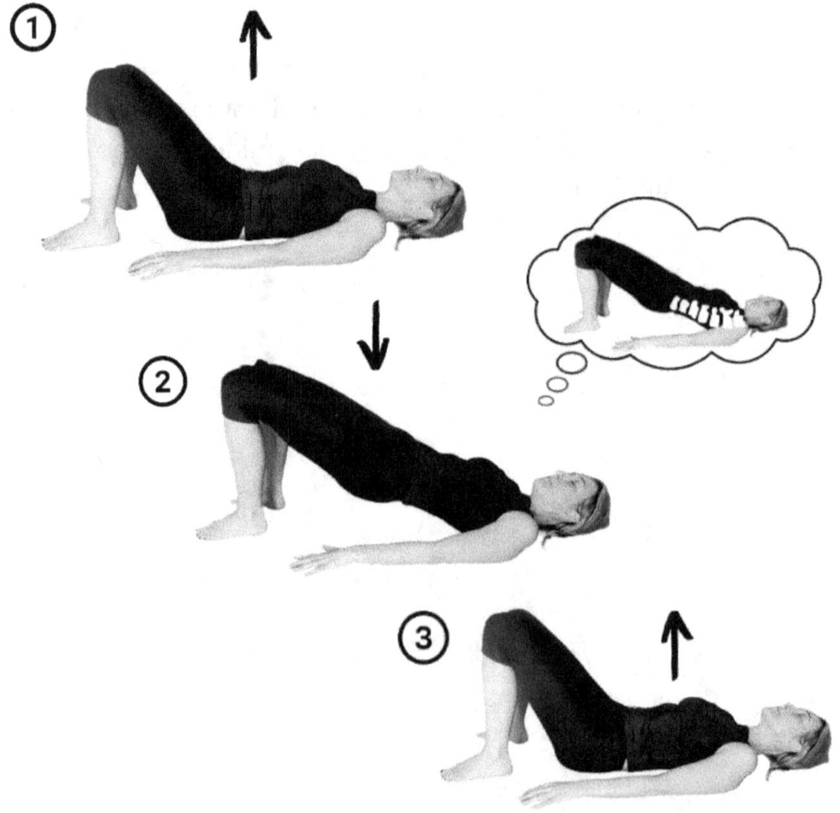

Perform the movement 15 times x 3 times

Position yourself with your back on the floor, arms stretched along your sides and knees bent. Inhale and lift your pelvis upward.

As you perform the exercise contract your glutes, visualize your inner strength and mentally repeat, "Each contraction brings me closer to my goal. I am strong, I am determined."

Hold the position for a few long breaths

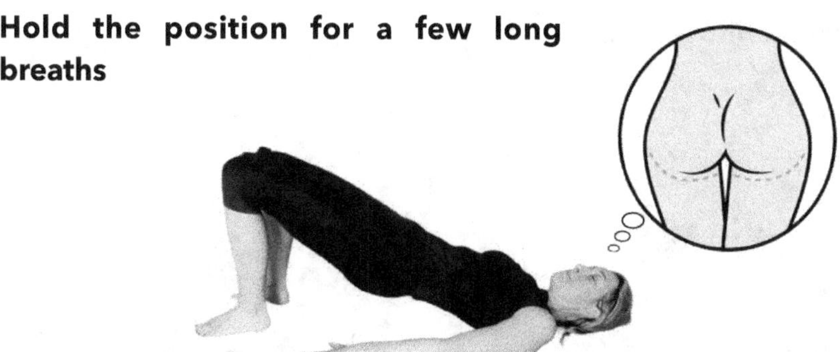

Position yourself with your back on the floor, and your hands behind the back of your head, Exhale and lift your shoulders off the floor. As you perform the exercise contract your abs, visualize your inner strength and mentally repeat, "Every effort is a
step toward wellness."

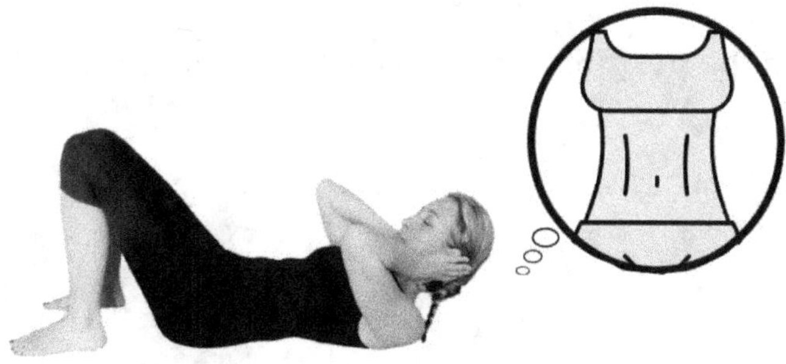

Hold the position for a few long breaths

Position yourself with your back on the floor, and your hands behind the back of your head, Exhale and lift your shoulders off the floor. (Figure 1)

To intensify the exercise, bring your elbows closer to your knees and contract your abs and glutes. (Figure 2)

Perform the movement 15 times x 3 times

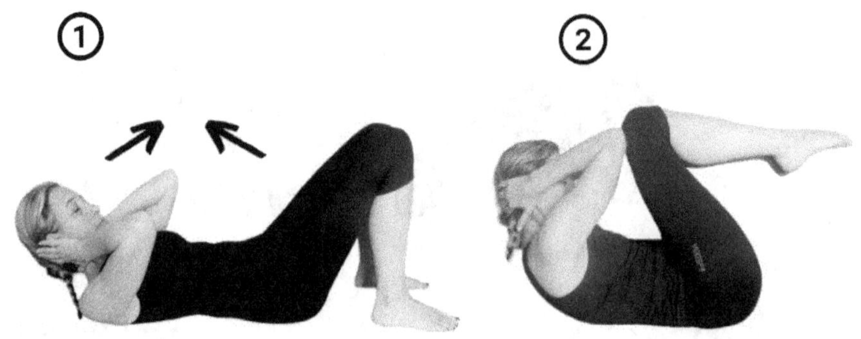

Exercise 5

As you perform the exercise contract your abs and glutes, visualize your inner strength and mentally repeat, "I am capable, I am good and I am important."

Hold the position for a few long breaths

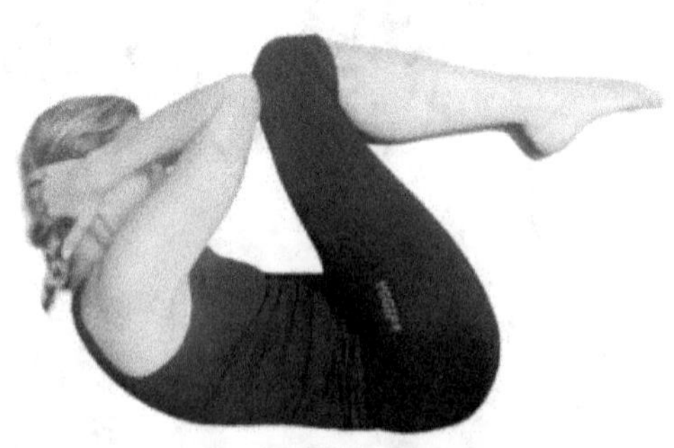

The boat pose in all its variations (see figures opposite), also known as "Navasana" in yoga, is critically important for releasing tension and gaining confidence by activating all the muscles in the body.

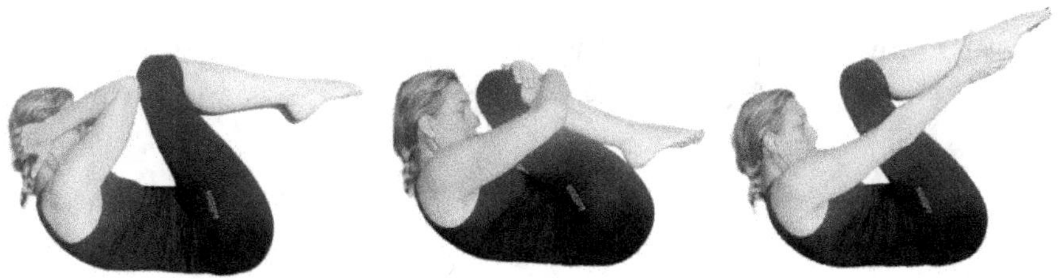

Full Muscle Activation:

The boat pose engages all major muscle groups, including abdominals, hip flexors, back and leg muscles. This comprehensive muscle activation helps to strengthen and tone the body in a balanced way o.

Dissolution of Tensions:

Maintaining the boat position stretches and strengthens the spine, releasing accumulated tension in the lower back and shoulders. Activating the abdominal muscles also helps stabilize the core, relieving stress on the back.

Improvement of Posture:

Regular practice of this exercise improves posture, reducing the risk of pain related to poor posture. Better posture contributes to greater self-confidence and a more solid physical presence.

Increased Security:

Challenging oneself to maintain the boat position, which requires balance and strength, can increase personal confidence. Achieving and maintaining balance in this position can convey a sense of control and mastery of one's body.

Stress Release:

Like many yoga postures, the boat encourages breath and body awareness. This focus helps reduce mental stress and promote a state of inner calm.

Promotion of Flexibility and Stability:

Boat exercise not only increases strength but also improves flexibility and stability, crucial elements for a balanced and healthy body.

In summary, boat exercise is an effective tool for releasing physical tension, improving overall muscle strength and gaining more confidence. Practicing this posture regularly can lead to significant physical and mental benefits, contributing to holistic well-being.

Keep this information in mind whenever you practice these exercises.

In somatic therapy, it is important to be aware of what you are doing to guide your mind and body in the direction of weight loss and greater flexibility and well-being.

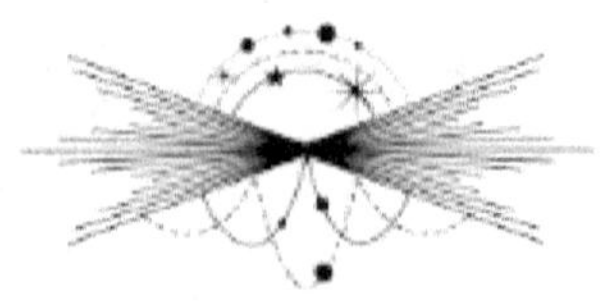

Position yourself sitting on the floor with your back straight and legs bent. Bring your left elbow past your right knee. (Figure 1)

Then bring the right elbow past the left knee. (Figure 2).

Torso twisting in somatic yoga is important to release muscle tension in the back and hips, improve circulation and stimulate internal organs, aiding digestion and reducing swelling. This movement can improve the pelvic area, releasing the body from tension and increasing freedom of sexual expression. Practice these twists with awareness and positive thoughts.

Perform the movement 15 times x 3 times

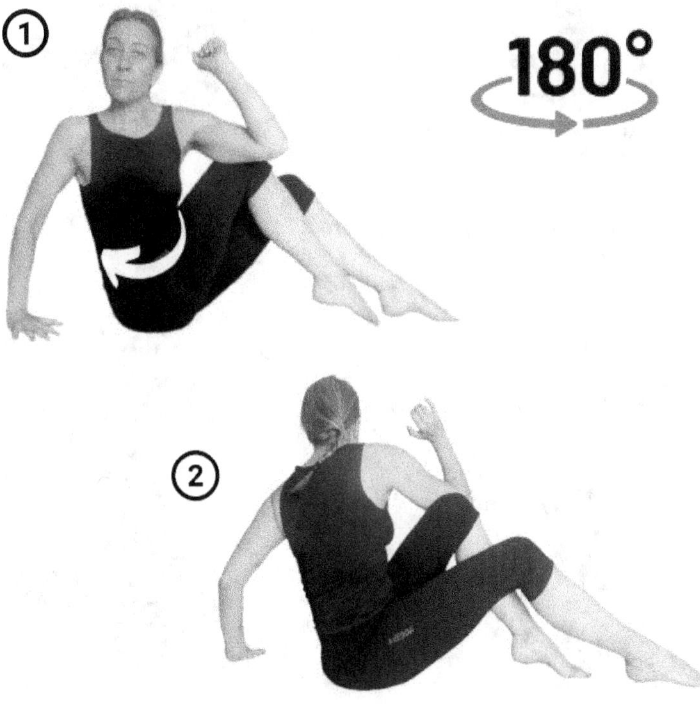

Sit comfortably with the spine erect. Keep your shoulders relaxed. Bring your hand to the opposite shoulder and rest your other hand on your elbow. (Figure 1)

Push the elbow outward focusing on the fluency of the movement. The gaze is directed behind the shoulder. (Figure 2) Practice these twists with awareness and positive thoughts.

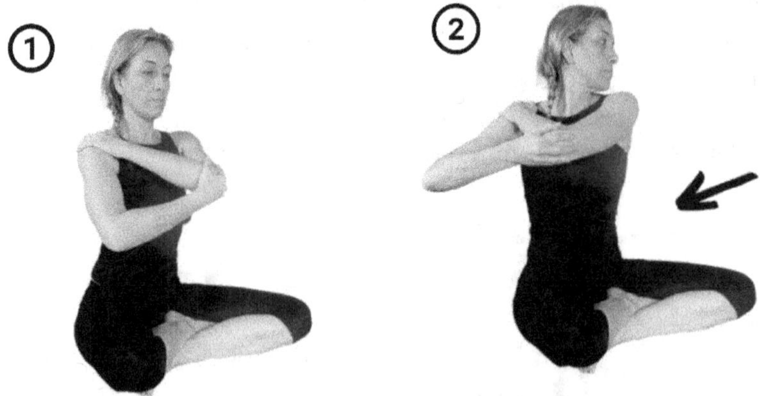

Hold the position for a few long breaths

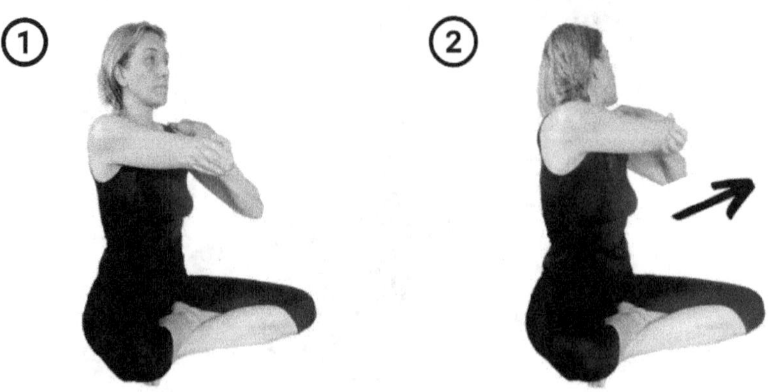

Repeat from the opposite side

Bend your torso forward, extending your arms in front of you, and rest your forehead on the ground.

Child's posture helps overcome trauma by releasing tension in the back and legs, which are often affected by emotional stress. This posture promotes a sense of safety and security, which is essential for coping with traumatic experiences. By relieving chronic tension related to feelings of insecurity and prolonged stress, child's pose helps the body find deep balance and relaxation.

Remain in this position a few minutes

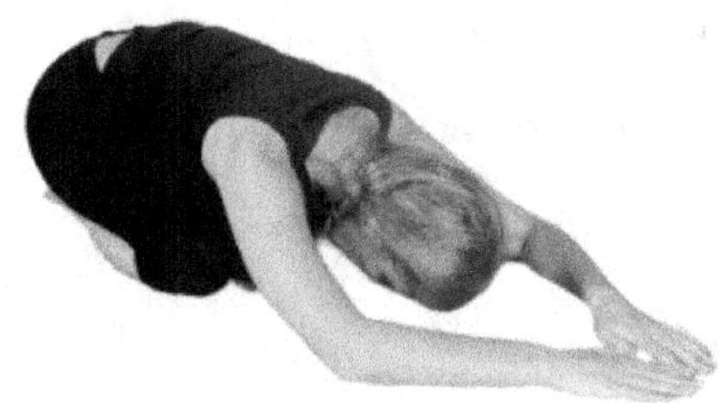

Phrase of the Day

To be repeated several times throughout the day:

"Change is never painful. Only resistance to change is." - Buddha

Gratification

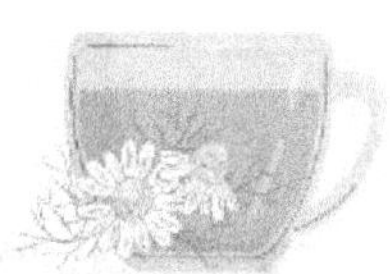

Drink herbal tea in a peaceful place where no one can disturb you.

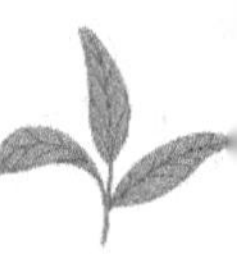

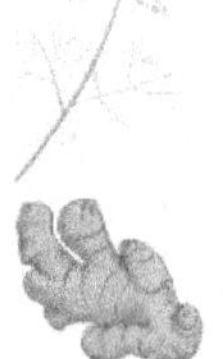

Ingredients:

- 1 tablespoon of dried green tea leaves
- 1 tablespoon of dried peppermint leaves
- 1 tablespoon of fennel seeds
- 1 teaspoon grated ginger root
- 2 cups of water

Instructions:

1. In a teapot, combine green tea leaves, peppermint leaves, fennel seeds and grated ginger root.

2. Bring 2 cups of water to a boil.

3. Pour the boiling water over the herbs in the teapot.

4. Cover and let steep for 5-10 minutes.

5. Strain the herbal tea to remove the herbs.

6. Pour into a cup and enjoy the hot herbal tea.

Benefits of Herbs Used:

Green Tea: Rich in antioxidants and compounds that can increase metabolism and promote fat burning.

Peppermint: Aids digestion and reduces appetite, promoting weight control.

Fennel Seeds: Support digestion, reduce bloating and improve metabolism function.

Ginger: Stimulates metabolism, improves digestion and has thermogenic properties that can aid in weight loss.

This herbal slimming herbal tea is a healthy drink that can support your weight loss efforts by improving metabolism and digestion.

Position yourself sitting on the floor with your elbows resting on the ground. Keep your back straight and perform the bicycle movement by rotating your legs clockwise. Perform the exercise tenderly with your gaze forward and your abdominal muscles contracted.

Perform the movement 15 times x 3 times, clockwise

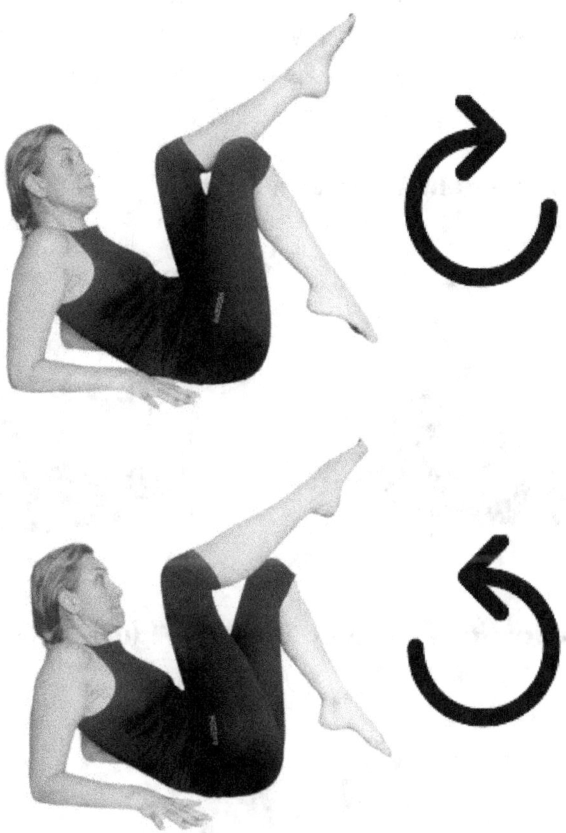

Perform the movement 15 times x 3 times, counterclockwise

Position yourself with your back resting on the floor, keep your knees flexed and grasp them with both hands. Keep your gaze upward. Inhale deeply. (Figure 1)

Exhale and bring the head toward the knees, activating the abdominals, until the lungs are completely empty. (Figure 2)

Listen to your abdominal muscles contract and your arms do strength as you perform the exercise. Coordination is an important aspect of somatic practice. Knowing which muscles to use and coordinating movements correctly is a way to be in control of your body and thus of your actions. Decide to be the master of your movements and do not let fatigue overwhelm you.

Perform the movement 15 times x 3 times

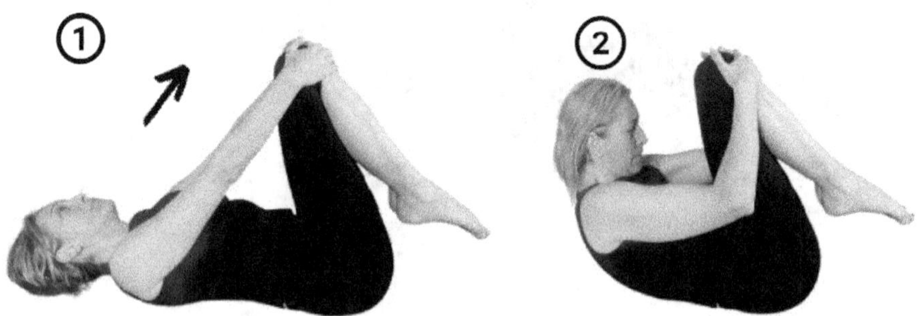

Hold the position for a few long breaths (Figure 3)

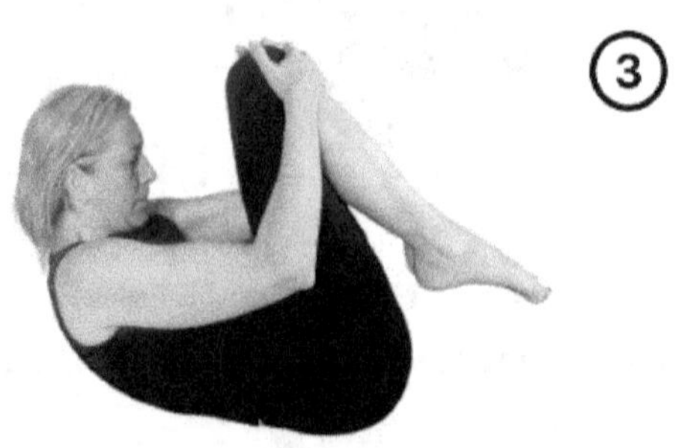

Position yourself on the floor with your back curved and your arms hugging your knees. Keep your head close to your knees. Keep your eyes closed. Listen to your body locked in this reassuring and protective position. Imagine your body as the safe house in which you can always take refuge. (Figure 1)

Hold the position for a few long breaths

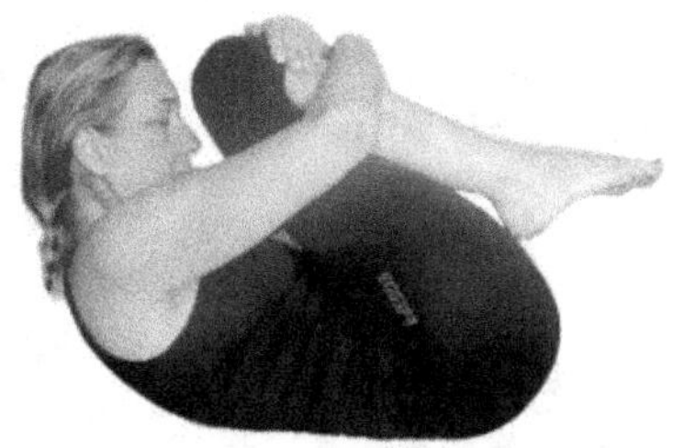

Get into the closed position and exhale. (Figure 1)

Inhale and extend your legs skyward, stretch your hands toward your ankles and lift your gaze and shoulders upward. (Figure 2)

Perform the movement 15 times x 3 times

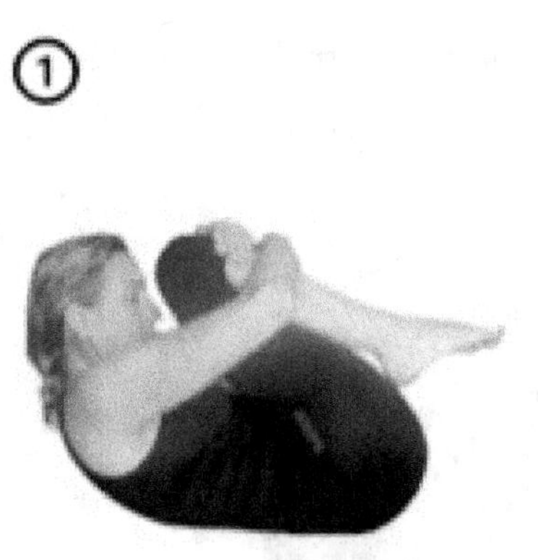

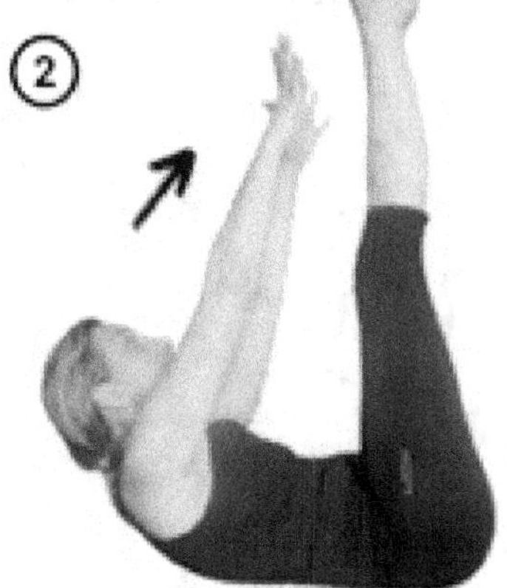

Position yourself with your back resting on the floor, grasp your knees with your hands. Feel the weight of your body on the floor. (Figure 1). Exhale and pull your knees toward your chest. Feel your back lengthen and your lungs empty. (Figure 2)

Imagine with each movement that you feel light and lucid. Look confidently ahead of you. See the world before you from a new perspective.

Perform the movement 15 times x 3 times

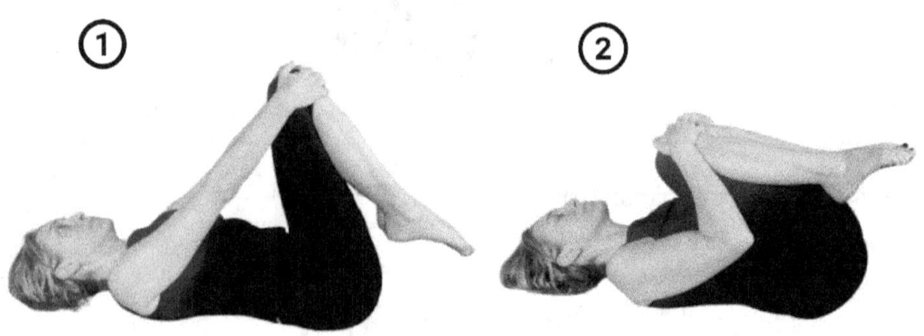

Hold the position for a few long breaths (Figure 3)

Imagine a sunny, warm sky filling the room.

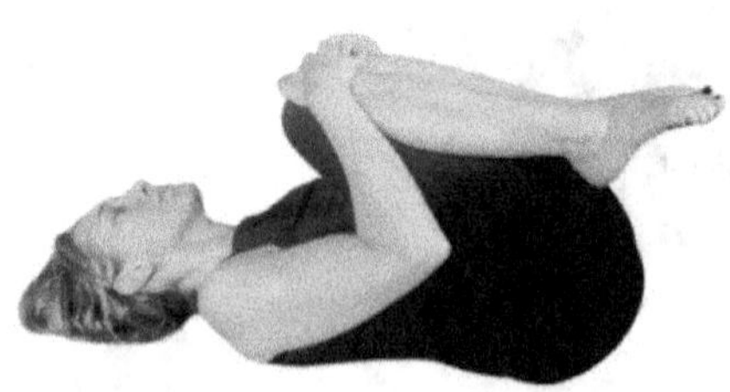

Get into the sitting position with your eyes closed. Take long breaths and imagine that you are safe. In a bright place full of radiance.

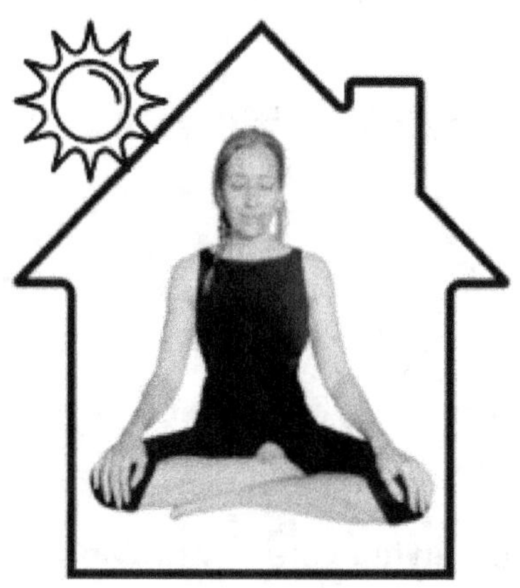

Phrase of the Day

To be repeated several times throughout the day:

""The body achieves what the mind believes in.""

Gratification

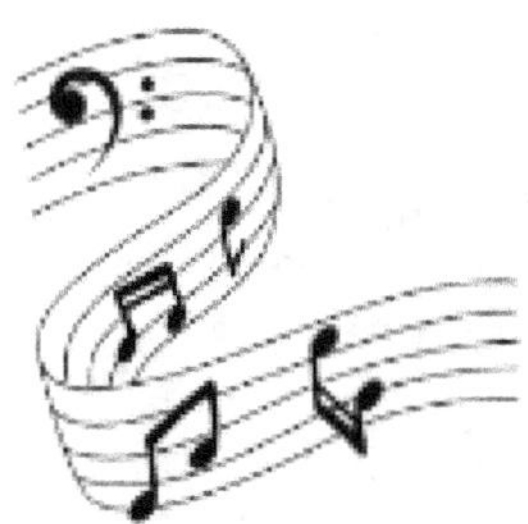

Listen to a song you really like in a quiet place and reflect on the emotions it stirs in you.

Music therapy uses the power of music to promote physical, emotional and mental well-being. In the context of weight loss, music therapy can play a crucial role in reducing stress, improving mood and providing motivation. In addition, music can help unlock trauma and mental barriers that often prevent long-term success in weight-loss diets.

Benefits of Music Therapy in Weight Loss:

Stress Reduction:

Relaxing music can reduce levels of the stress hormone cortisol, which is often associated with the accumulation of abdominal fat.

Improvement of Mood:

Stimulating music can elevate mood and increase motivation, making it easier to follow a diet and exercise program.

Promoting Relaxation:

Listening to calm music can help improve sleep and overall relaxation, which are essential for effective weight management.

Unlocking Trauma and Mental Barriers:

Music can evoke emotions and memories, helping to process and release past traumas that could negatively affect eating habits.

Types of Music to Choose:

Classical Music:

Examples: pieces by composers such as Bach, Mozart and Beethoven.

Benefits: Reduces stress and promotes relaxation. Ideal for moments of meditation and reflection.

Ambient music:

Examples: Artists such as Brian Eno, Ludovico Einaudi.

Benefits: Creates a quiet and peaceful environment, useful for meditation and mindfulness.

Instrumental Music:

Examples: Movie soundtracks, music by artists such as Yanni or Enya.

Benefits: Stimulates imagination and helps release pent-up emotions.

New Age music:

Examples: Artists such as Enya, Deep Forest.

Benefits: Promotes relaxation and inner connection, useful for yoga or meditation sessions.

Motivational Pop Music:

Examples: Energetic and motivational songs by artists such as Beyoncé, Imagine Dragons.

Benefits: Increases energy and motivation, perfect for training sessions.

How to Use Music Therapy:

Relaxation Sessions: Listen to soothing music during daily relaxation moments to reduce stress and improve mood.

Guided Meditation: Use ambient music tracks during meditation to enhance concentration and relaxation.

Exercise Fitness: Create a playlist of motivational music to accompany workout sessions, increasing energy and stamina.

Moments of Reflection: Listening to classical or instrumental music during moments of personal reflection to help process emotions and trauma.

Music provides an important and enjoyable life support. Choosing the right music can make a big difference in the success of the weight loss journey.

Practical application:

Listen to a soothing track of ambient or classical music while lying comfortably with your eyes closed, or sitting, focusing on the feelings that emerge. If the flow of thoughts becomes too painful, stop the music and take a moment to breathe deeply and regain calm. This gradual approach helps unlock mental barriers without overloading emotions.

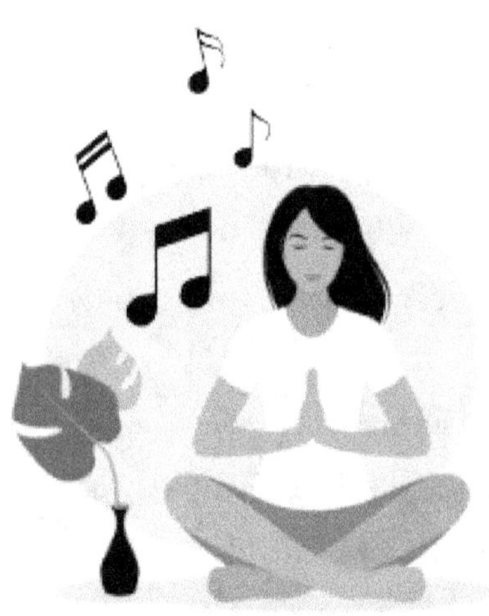

Exercise 1

Sit cross-legged and bring your hand to the opposite shoulder and rest your other hand on your elbow. Breathe slowly, paying attention to the sensations in your body. (Figure 1)

Push your elbow upward with your hand while focusing on shoulder looseness. (Figure 2)

Perform the movement 15 times x 3 times, with the left arm

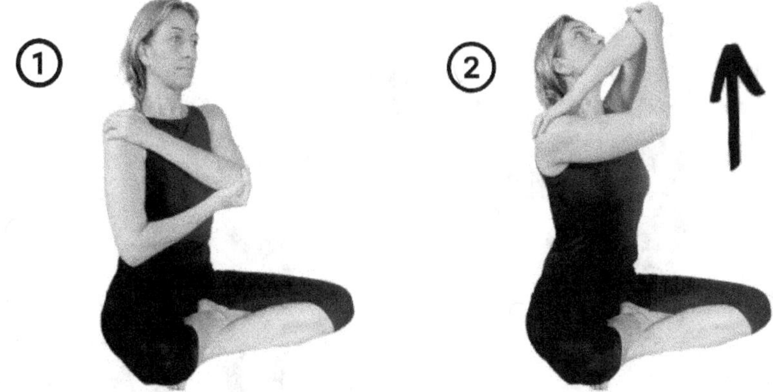

Perform the movement 15 times x 3 times, with the right arm

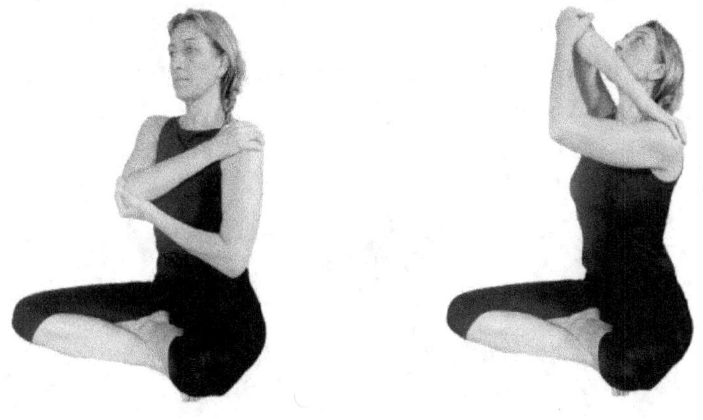

Position yourself in a quadrupedal position, with your hands firmly on the ground and your back straight. Feel the ground beneath you supporting you. (Figure 1)

Exhale and do a push-up with your arms, bringing your forehead down to the floor and keeping your back straight. (Figure 2)

You are strong and your arms are able to support you. Feel the muscles in your arms working for you.

Perform the movement 15 times x 3 times

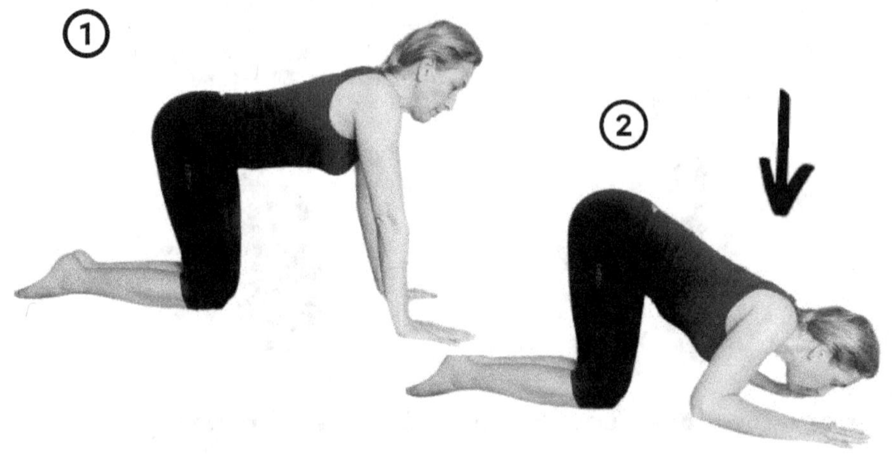

Hold the position with your elbows slightly raised off the ground, for a few long breaths (Figure 3)

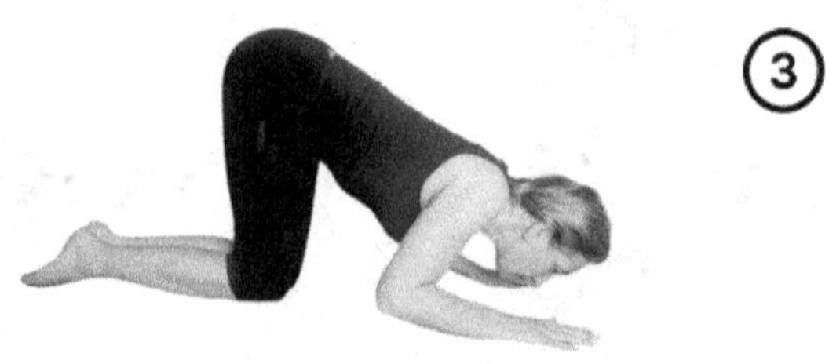

Position yourself sitting on the floor your arms flexed and feet raised. Arms are stretched out in front of you. Gaze upward. (Figure 1)

Exhale and lift your shoulders off the ground. Extend your hands upward. (Figure 2)

Often the belly is a place where fat accumulates. Underneath the fat are abdominal muscles that if reactivated can reduce the waistline and relieve back and hip pain.

Perform the movement 15 times x 3 times

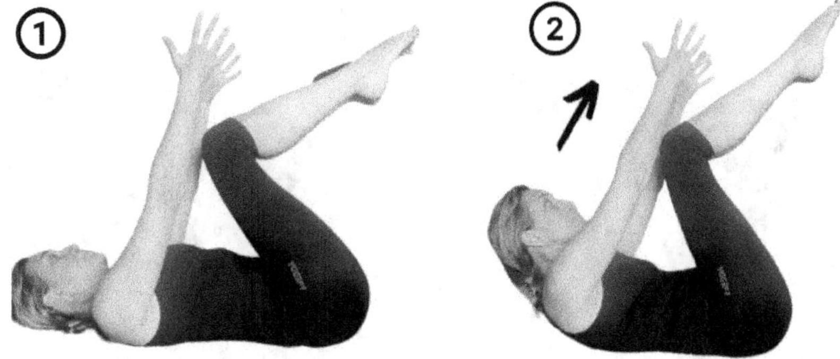

Exercise 5

Hold the position for a few long breaths, imagining the abdominal muscles contracted and active. (Figure 3)

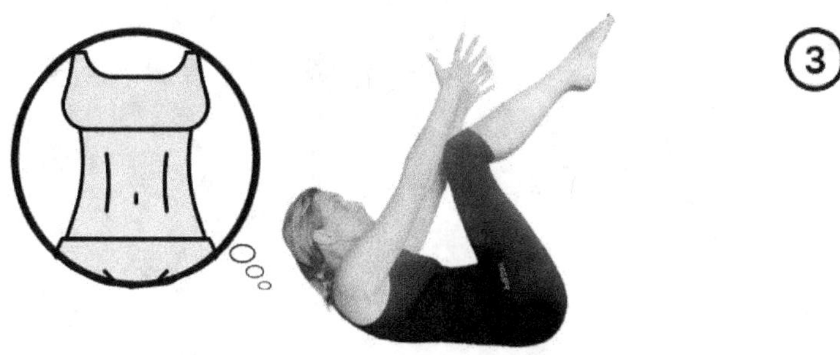

Position yourself in quadrupedal position, with your hands firmly on the ground and your back straight. (Figure 1)

Exhale and do a push-up with your arms, bringing your forehead down to the floor and keeping your back straight. (Figure 2)

Inhale and putting strength in your arms and legs go into the mountain position. (Figure 3)

Perform the movement 15 times x 3 times

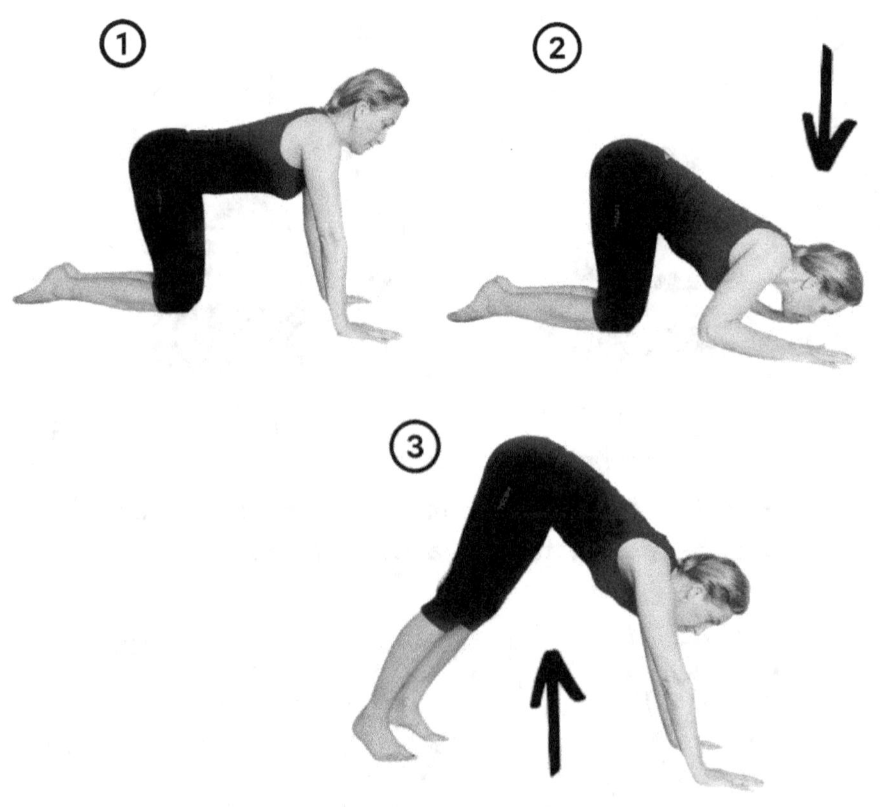

The Mountain posture is a very powerful posture. You should practice this exercise every morning and every evening because it has the following benefits:

Stability and Concentration: The Mountain pose requires you to maintain a stable balance, which helps improve concentration and body awareness. This physical stability can translate into mental stability, helping you overcome negative thoughts and mental barriers that hinder your weight loss journey.

Body and Mind Alignment: This posture helps realign the spine and improve posture, promoting a feeling of grounding and centering. A well-aligned body allows for a clearer, more focused mind, facilitating more conscious decisions about diet and exercise.

Breath Awareness: Focusing on the breath while practicing Tadasana helps calm the mind and reduce stress. Stress is often a contributing factor to weight gain, so learning to manage it through mindful breathing is crucial.

Muscle Activation: Although it sounds simple, the Mountain pose involves several muscle groups, including the abdominals, legs, and back muscles. Keeping these muscles active helps improve muscle tone and increase metabolism, thus supporting weight loss.

Confidence in **Yourself**: Standing with an upright posture and mindful presence can increase self-confidence. Feeling more confident about one's body and abilities is a key element in facing the challenges of weight loss with determination and positivity.

Exercise 7

The Mountain pose also known as Tadasana, is one of the fundamental postures of yoga. It is not just a physical exercise, but a powerful tool for cultivating a strong and resilient mind, essential for breaking down mental barriers and promoting a healthy and sustainable weight loss path.

Distribute the weight: Balance the weight of the body evenly on both soles of the feet.

Align the body: Lift the knees, contract the thigh muscles slightly and keep the legs straight but not stiff. Activate the abdominals by pulling the belly button toward the spine.

Stretch the spine: Imagine you are being pulled upward from the top of your head. Keep your shoulders relaxed and your arms along your sides, palms facing forward.

Hold the position for a few long breaths.

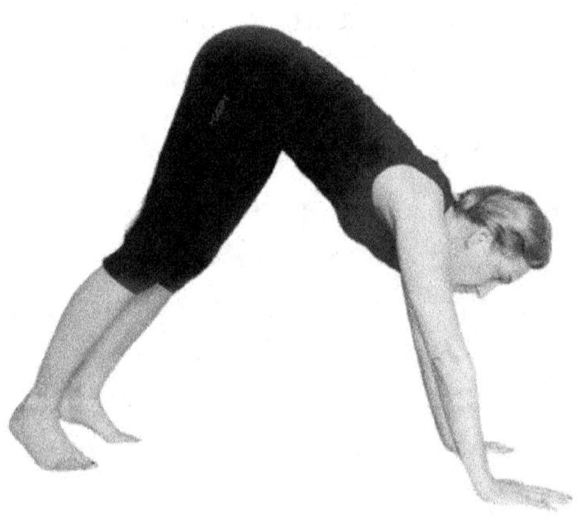

Rest your hands on your belly and breathe deeply, feeling the rise and fall of the abdomen.

Your belly is like a balloon that inflates and deflates. You should feel your hands rise as you inhale (Figure 1) and lower as you exhale. (Figure 2)

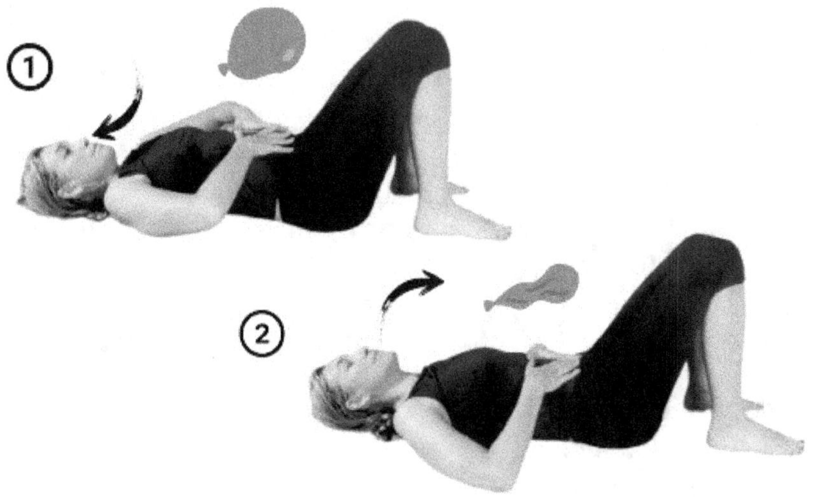

Phrase of the Day

To be repeated several times throughout the day:

"Motivation gets you started. Habit keeps you going." - Jim Ryun

Gratification

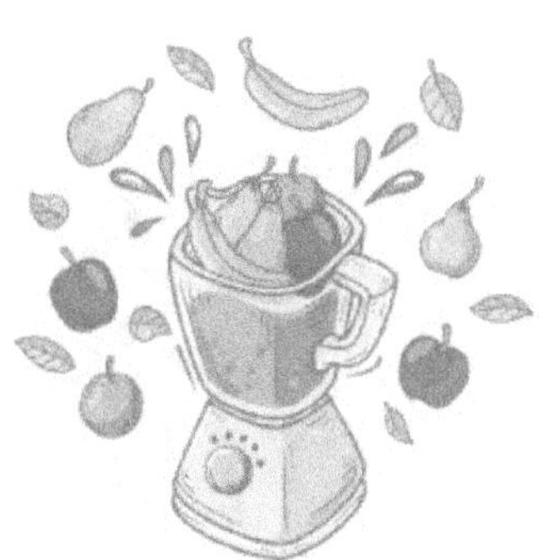

Make a diet smoothie. Taking your time to choose the ingredients. Prepare it with love and enjoy it in a quiet place.

Ingredients:

- 1 cup of fresh spinach

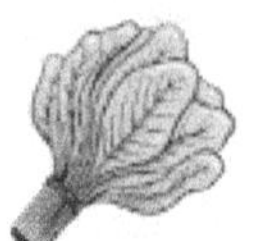

- 1 green apple, peeled and cut into pieces

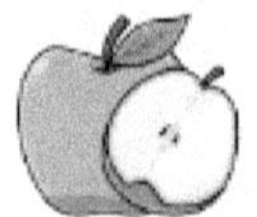

- 1/2 cucumber, cut into pieces

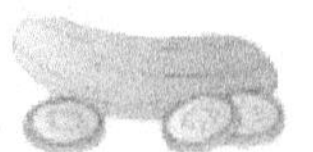

- 1/2 ripe avocado

- 1 cup of coconut water or natural water

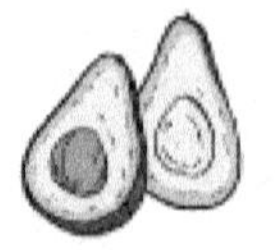

- Juice of 1/2 lemon

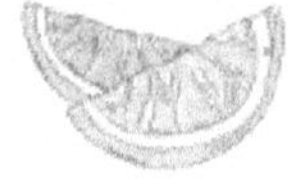

- Ice cubes (optional)

Instructions:

1. Place the spinach, apple, cucumber and avocado in the blender.

2. Add coconut water or natural water.

3. Squeeze fresh lemon juice.

4. Blend until smooth and homogeneous.

5. Add ice cubes for a cooler smoothie, if desired.

6. Pour into a glass and enjoy immediately.

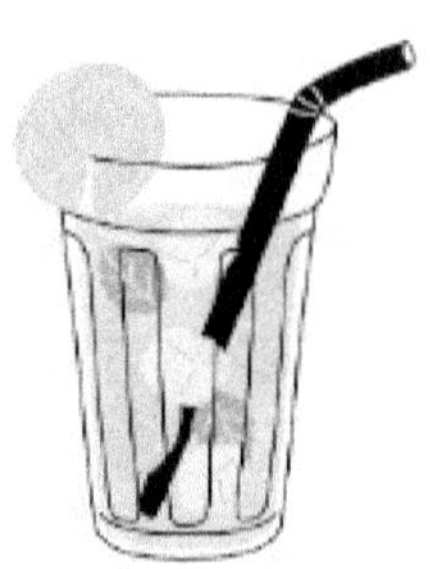

This smoothie is rich in fiber, vitamins and minerals, ideal for a balanced diet.

Exercise 1

Position yourself sitting on the floor with arms flexed and feet raised. Arms are stretched out in front of you. Gaze upward. (Figure 1)

Exhale and lift your shoulders off the ground. Try to reach your feet with your hands. (Figure 2)

Perform the movement 15 times x 3 times

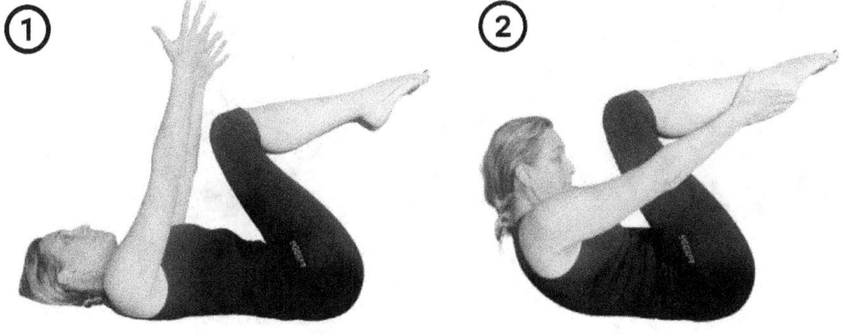

Exercise 2

Hold the position for a few long breaths, imagining the abdominal muscles contracted and active. (Figure 3)

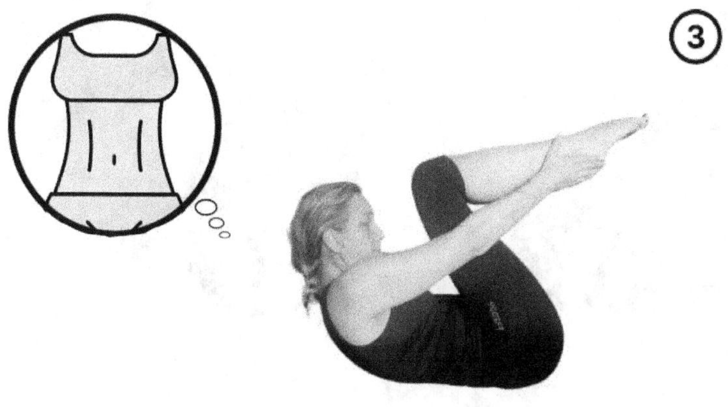

Stand on your back and grasp your heels with your hands. (Figure 1)

Rock forward on your back carrying your weight on your glutes. The abdominals are contracted. (Figure 2)

Perform the rolling motion 15 times x   3 times

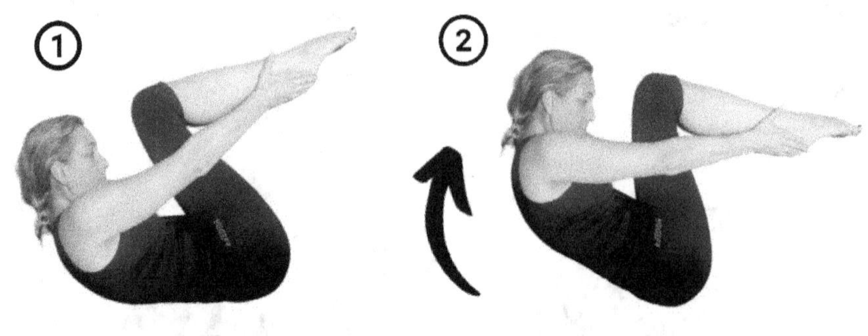

Stand on your back and grasp your heels with your hands. (Figure 1)

Rock back on your back by carrying your weight on your shoulders. The abdominals are contracted. (Figure 2)

Perform the movement 15 times x 3 times

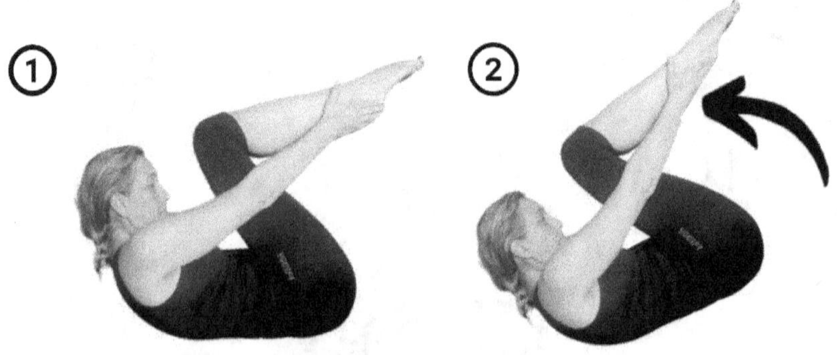

Read this section before proceeding to the next exercise.

Mobility of the neck and shoulders is essential to eliminate mental barriers, because these areas of the body tend to accumulate tension due to stress and unprocessed emotions. When the neck and shoulders are stiff, not only do you experience physical pain, but you may also feel mental blocks, as if thoughts and emotions are trapped.

Accumulated tension: The neck and shoulders are particularly sensitive to stress. Stressful situations and daily worries can cause muscle tension, leading to stiffness and pain.

Fat: Fat tends to accumulate in these areas due to a combination of stress, poor posture and lack of movement. Psychosomatically, accumulated fat in the shoulders and neck may be a signal from the body that it is trying to protect itself from heavy emotional loads.

Psychosomatic causes: Emotional stress and anxiety often manifest physically in these areas. Repressed emotions, such as anger or sadness, can result in chronic muscle tension. The body, in response to stress, may increase production of cortisol, the stress hormone, which contributes to fat accumulation.

Solutions

Mobility Exercises: Practice regular stretching and mobility exercises for the neck and shoulders. This helps release accumulated tension and improve circulation.

Relaxation Techniques: Use relaxation techniques such as deep breathing, yoga or meditation to reduce stress and muscle tension.

Body Awareness: Pay attention to how your body reacts to stressful situations. Learn to recognize and release tensions as they arise.

Reflection Questions

- What situations or emotions tend to cause tension in your neck and shoulders?

- Can you identify specific times when you have accumulated tension in these areas?

- What relaxation techniques have you found helpful in relieving tension in the past?

- How does movement and exercise affect your feelings of tension in your neck and shoulders?

- Have you noticed a correlation between your stress levels and fat accumulation in these areas?

Understanding these dynamics and taking action to improve neck and shoulder mobility can have a significant impact on your physical and mental well-being, helping you overcome mental barriers and promote holistic health.

Keep this information in mind whenever you practice somatic exercises. This will enable you to have a compassionate attitude toward your body and your tensions, helping you to release them.

Sit comfortably with your spine erect, and your legs crossed on the floor. Place your arms behind your head.   Inhale deeply, opening your chest. (Figure 1)

Exhale and close your elbows in front of you (Figure 2)

Perform the movement 15 times x 3 times

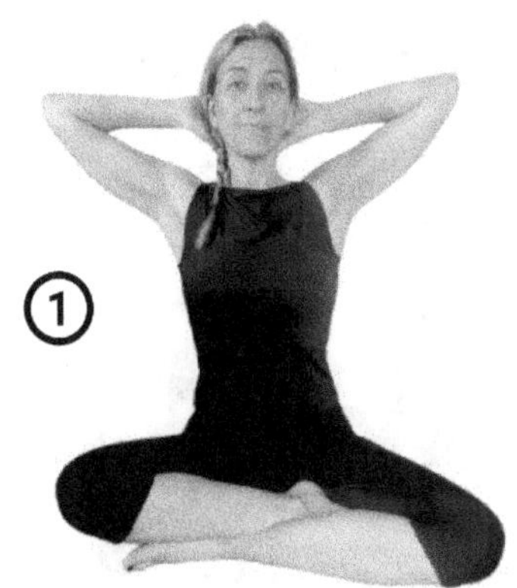
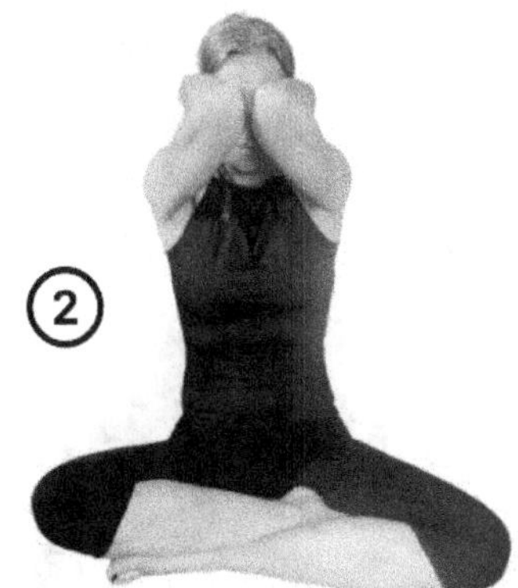

Sit comfortably with the spine erect. Keep your shoulders relaxed. Gently wrap your head with one hand and apply gentle pressure to the right. (Figure 1) Hold the position for a few breaths then repeat to the left. (Figure 2)

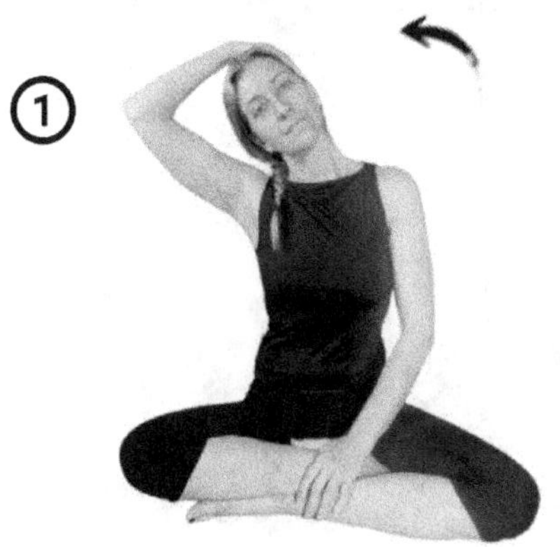
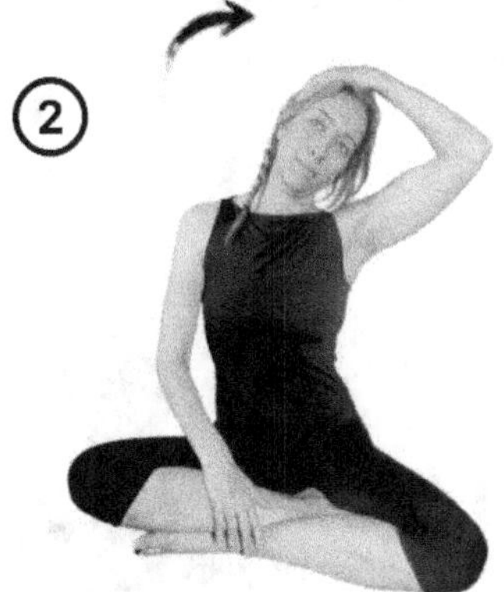

Position yourself sitting on the floor your arms flexed and feet raised. Arms are stretched out in front of you. Gaze upward. (Figure 1)

Exhale and perform a flexion by twisting the body to the right. Remember that twisting releases stress and tension. Listen to your body's sensations during the exercise. (Figure 2)

Perform the movement 15 times x 3 times to the right

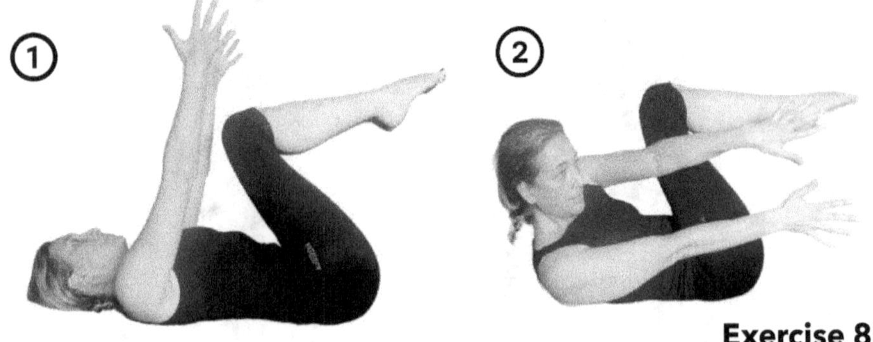

Position yourself sitting on the floor your arms flexed and feet raised. Arms are stretched out in front of you. Gaze upward. (Figure 1) Exhale and perform a flexion by twisting the body to the right. (Figure 2)

Perform the movement 15 times x 3 times to the left

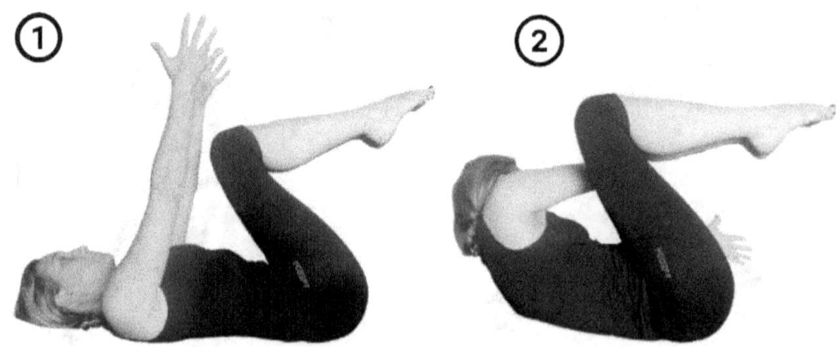

Hold the position to the right for a few long breaths

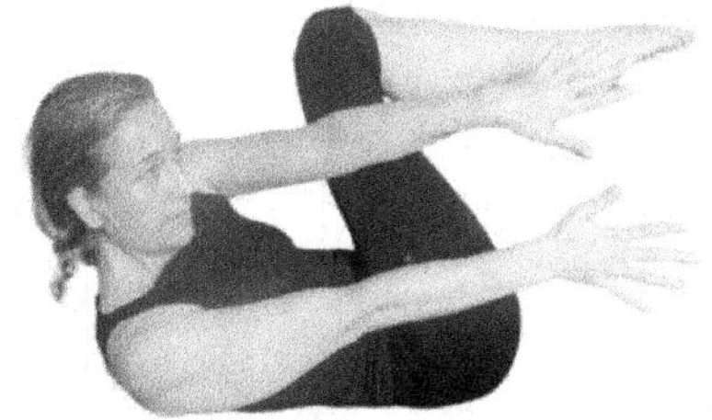

Hold the position to the left for a few long breaths

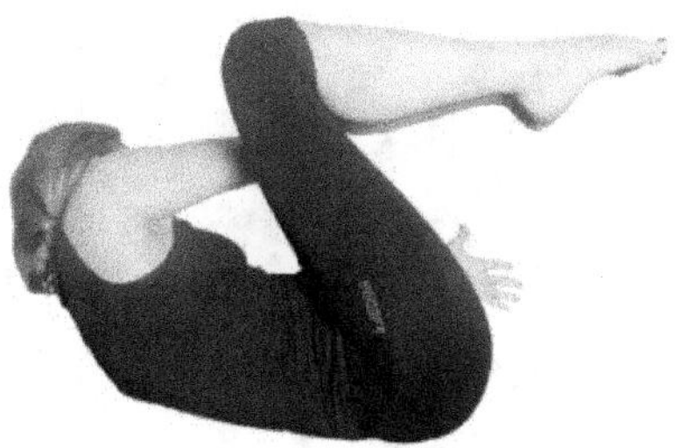

Perform the movement 15 times x 3 times alternating left and right push-ups

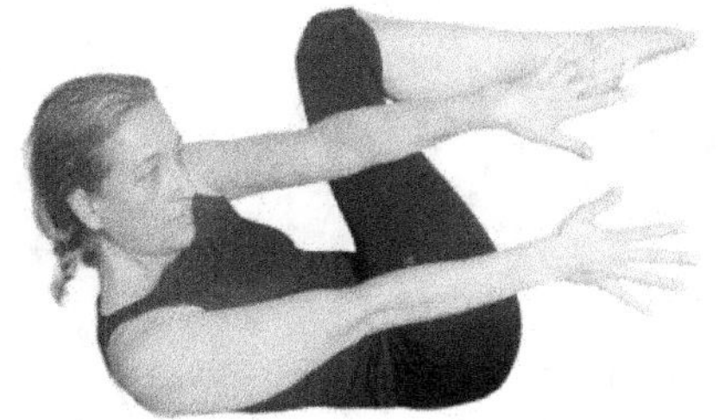

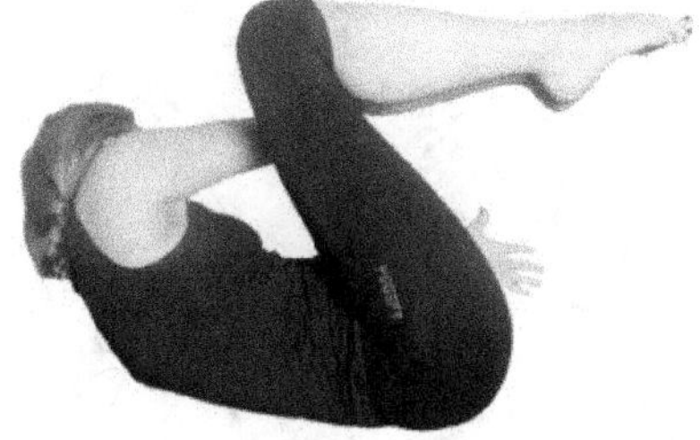

Bend your torso forward, extending your arms in front of you, and rest your forehead on the floor. Breathe deeply, allowing the body to relax completely.

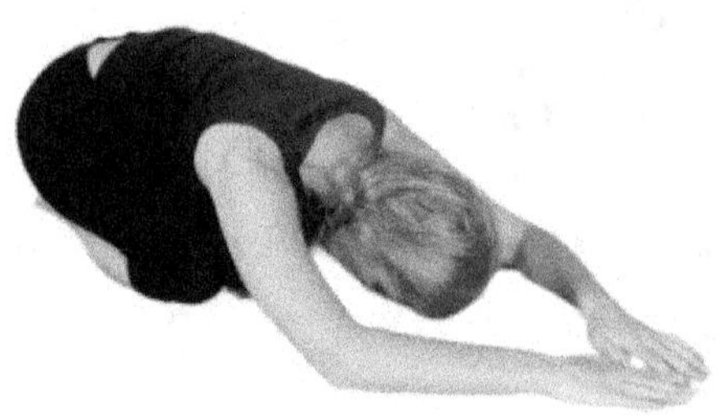

Phrase of the Day

To be repeated several times throughout the day:

"Discipline is the bridge between goals and results." - Jim Rohn

Gratification

Stand barefoot in the grass.

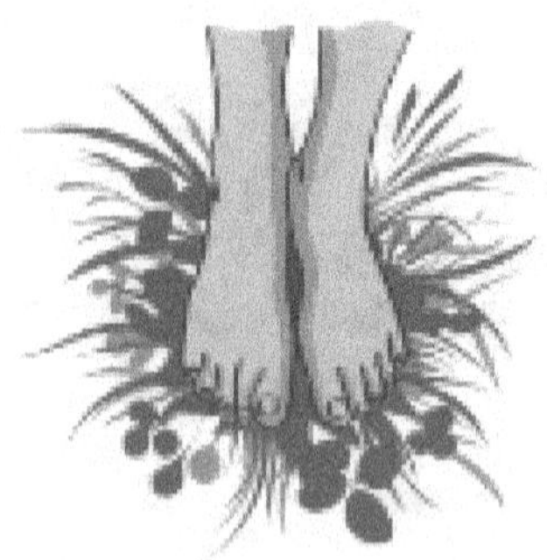

Origins of Grounding

The origins of grounding, or grounding, go back to the ancestral practices of cultures that lived in close harmony with nature. Our ancestors spent most of their time barefoot, allowing the body to absorb the energy of the earth. This habit improved their physical and mental well-being, a direct connection with the earth that has been rediscovered and scientifically studied for its many benefits.

Why Grounding is Useful

Grounding is beneficial because it helps reduce inflammation, relieve stress, improve sleep quality and increase a sense of balance and calm. These benefits result from direct skin contact with the earth's surface, which allows the exchange of free electrons between the body and the earth, balancing the body's electrical system and promoting overall health.

Grounding and Slimming

During a weight-loss journey, grounding can promote success in several ways. It helps keep a calm and focused mind, reducing stress and anxiety that often lead to poor and emotional food choices. In addition, grounding increases body awareness, allowing you to listen better to your body's signals and respond more effectively to physical needs.

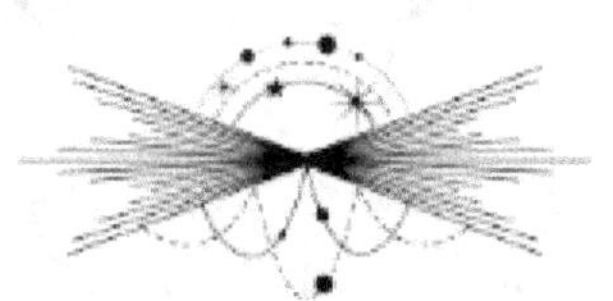

Exercise 1

Position yourself lying down with your back flat against the floor and your legs bent against your chest. Arms are stretched along your sides. Do an upward flexion of the hands and feet to loosen the joints. (Figure 1)

Make a downward flexion of the hands and feet. (Figure 2)

Perform the movement 15 times x 3 times

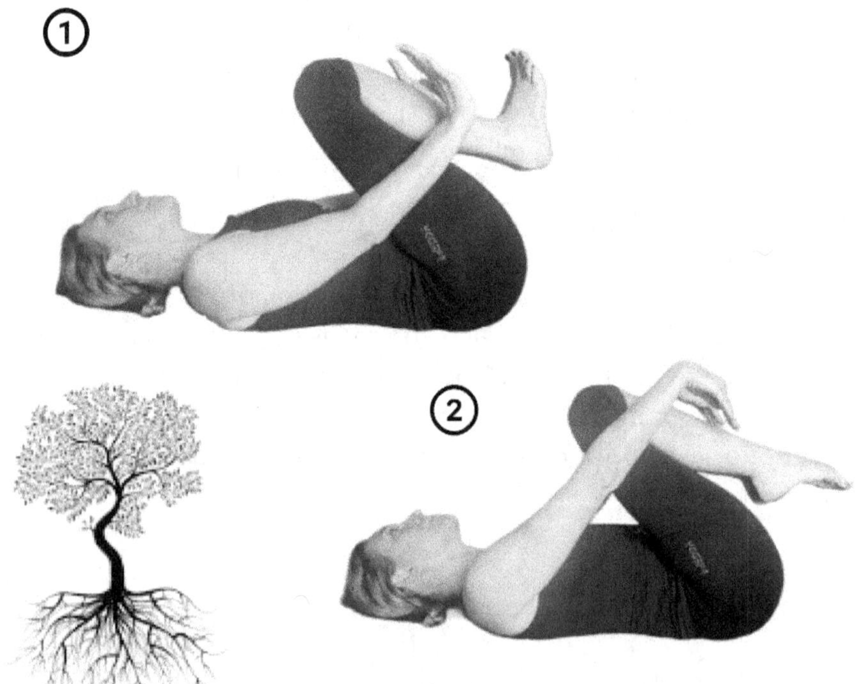

The feet are your roots, essential for the support and balance of the body. They connect you to the earth, providing stability and strength in every step you take. Nurturing and strengthening them is critical to maintaining proper posture and overall physical well-being.

Rotate hands and feet 15 times x 3 times, counterclockwise

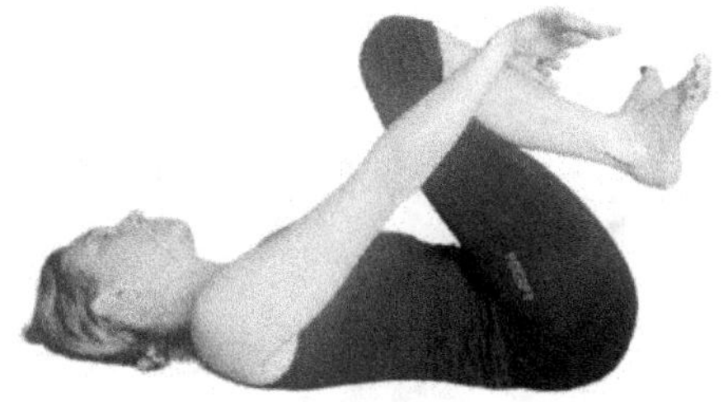

Rotate hands and feet 15 times x 3 times, clockwise

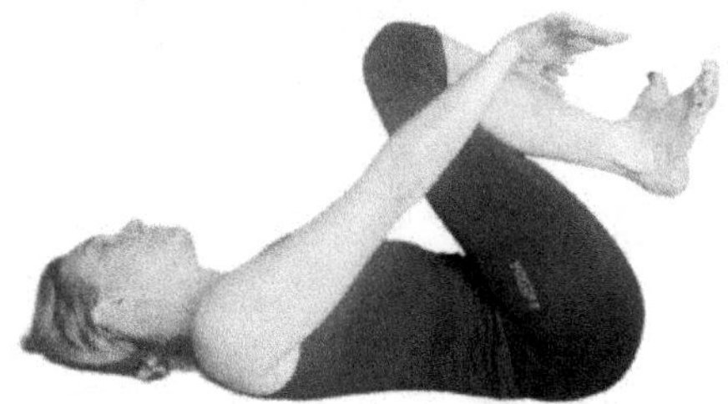

Exercise 3

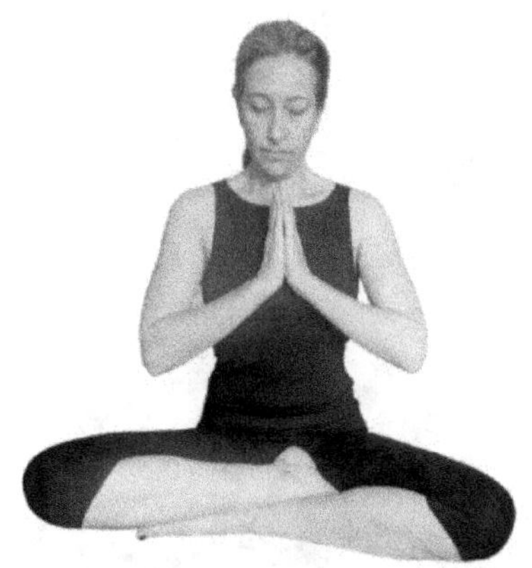

Sit with arms crossed and hands joined at the chest. Feel the energy flowing into your hands and feet and take long breaths.

Sit on the floor with your back straight and rotate your head left and right. Listen to the tendons in your neck stretch gently. Imagine that you are removing all the weights you are carrying from your shoulders.

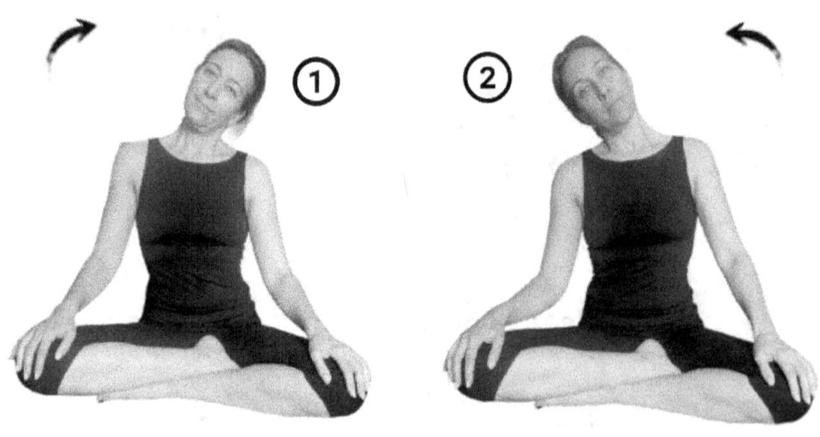

Sit on the floor with your back straight and lift your shoulders up and then down. Repeat the exercise until your shoulders and neck feel free and loose.

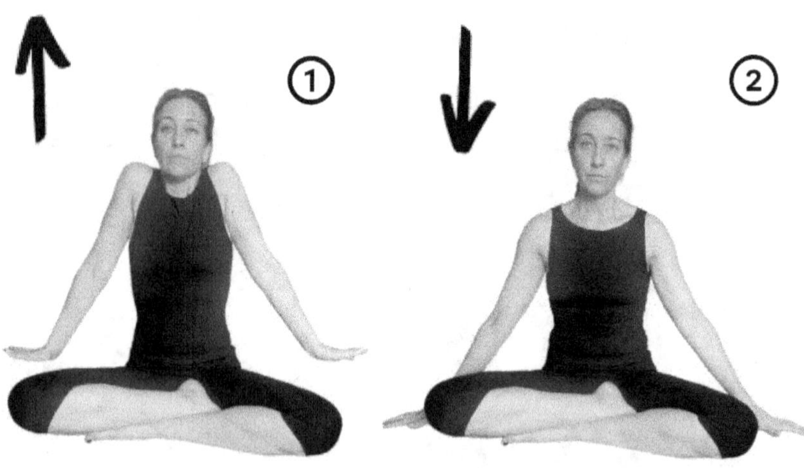

Sit on the floor with your back straight and rest your hands on your shoulders. Perform rotations with your arms, taking long breaths. Remember to reflect on the importance of shoulder and neck looseness, which we addressed in a previous chapter.

Rotate 15 times x 3 times, forward

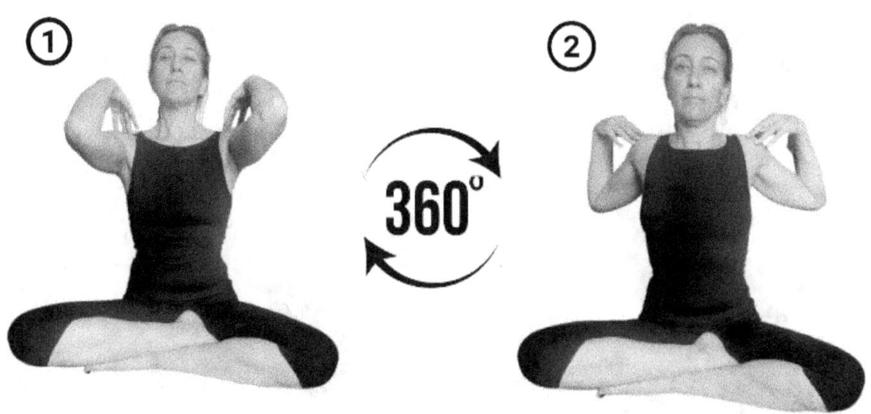

Rotate 15 times x 3 times, forward

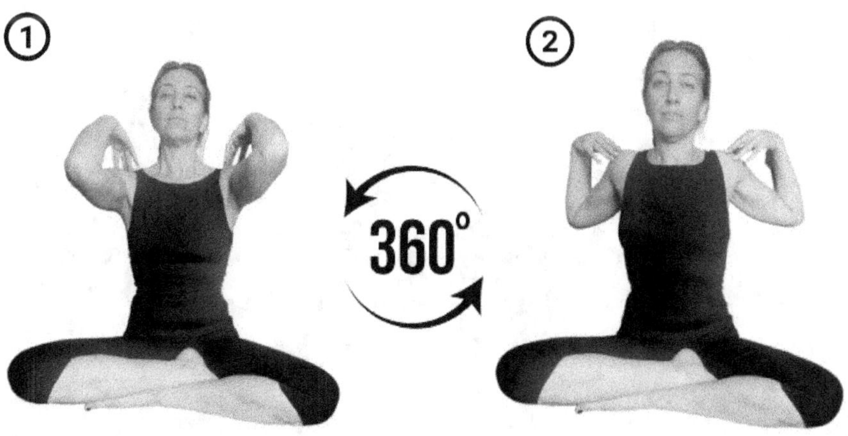

Sit on the floor with your back straight and apposite hands in front of you, holding your arms outstretched and looking forward. (Figure 1)

Exhale and perform an arm flexion until your elbows are brought to the floor. Keep your back straight and your gaze forward. (Figure 2)

Perform the movement 15 times x 3 times

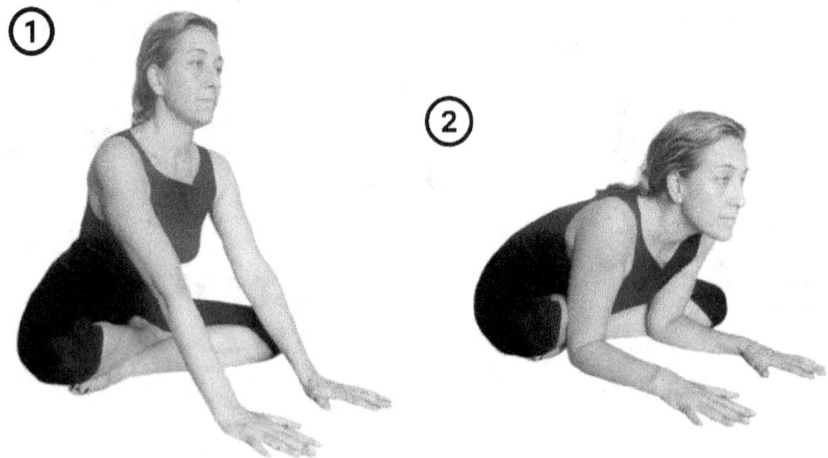

Hold the position for a few long breaths

Feel your belly swell and deflate and your arms support you firmly.

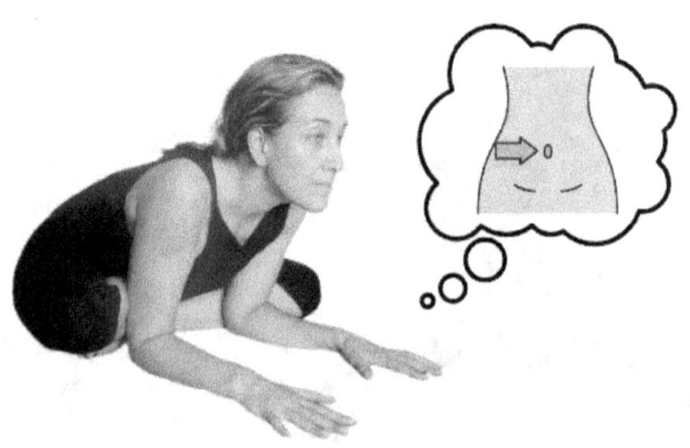

Intensify the previous exercise by performing a deeper push-up. Lower your gaze to the floor and keep your shoulders down.

Hold the position for a few long breaths

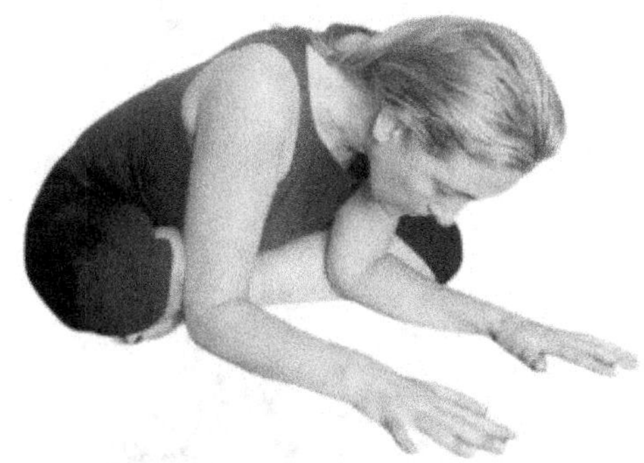

Exercise 9

With both hands wrap the back of your head and flex your head forward (Figure 1)·

Then painfully bring your head toward the floor by arching your back. (Figure 2)

Hold this position for a few long breaths.

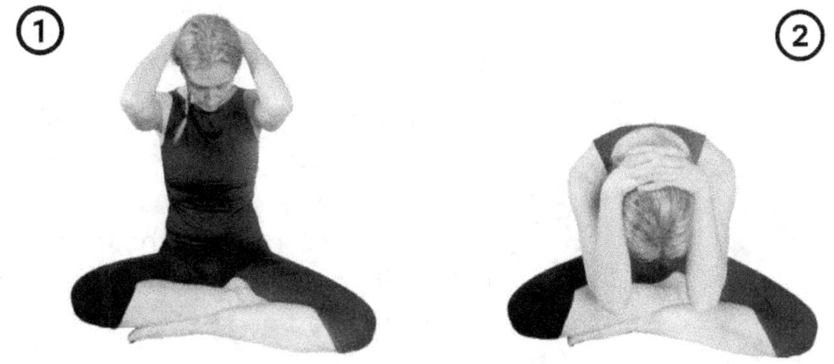

Get into the sitting position with your eyes closed.

Take long breaths and imagine a bright light enveloping your head and entering your body, filling it with energy and well-being.

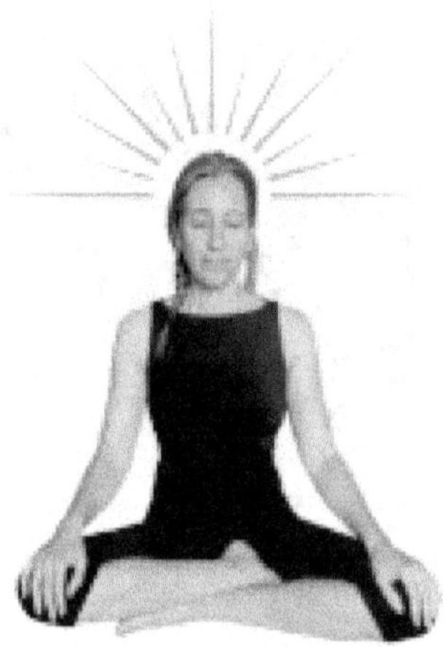

Phrase of the Day

To be repeated several times throughout the day:

"Your only limitation is the one you impose on your own mind." - *Napoleon Hill*

Gratification

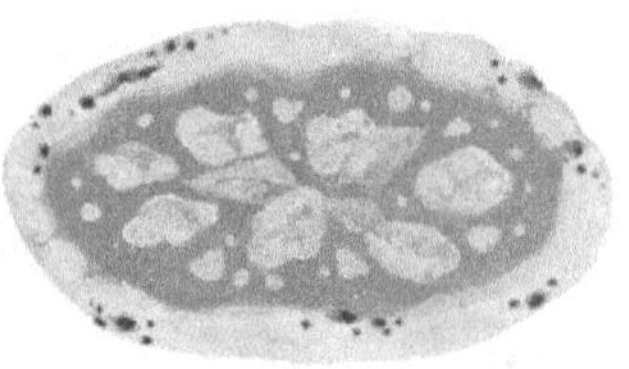

Reward yourself with a delicious dinner. Did you know that even if you want to lose weight, you can eat pizza? Find out the recipe for a light, digestible, low-calorie pizza on the next page.

Ingredients:

200g of lentil flour

50g wholemeal flour

1 teaspoon instant yeast

1 teaspoon salt

2 tablespoons of olive oil

200ml lukewarm water

200g of tomato puree

150g light mozzarella or low-fat cheese of your choice

Fresh vegetables to taste (peppers, zucchini, mushrooms, spinach)

Aromatic herbs (oregano, basil)

Salt and pepper to taste.

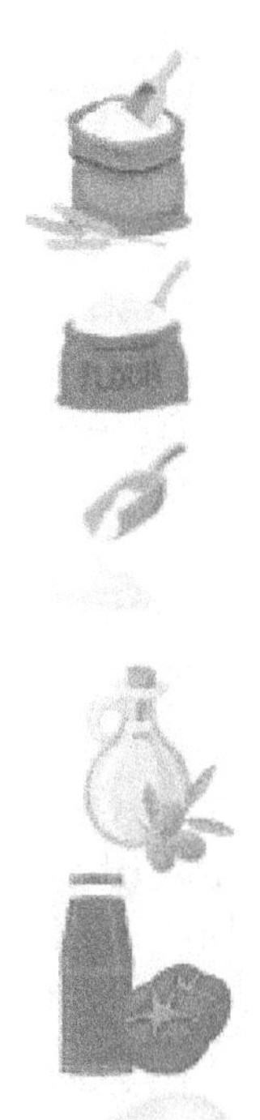

Dough preparation:

In a large bowl, mix the lentil flour, whole wheat flour, baking powder, and salt.

Add the olive oil and lukewarm water, mixing until smooth.

Knead the dough on a floured surface for about 5-7 minutes, until it becomes smooth and elastic.

Form a ball with the dough and let it rest covered with a damp cloth for 30 minutes.

Base preparation:

Preheat the oven to 220°C.

Roll out the dough on a lightly oiled baking sheet or covered with baking paper, forming a disk about 1 cm thick.

Seasoning:

Spread the tomato puree evenly over the dough.

Add light mozzarella or thinly sliced low-fat cheese.

Add the chopped fresh vegetables.

Sprinkle with herbs, salt and pepper to taste.

Cooking:

Bake the pizza in the preheated oven for about 15 to 20 minutes, until the base is golden and the cheese is melted and lightly browned.

Service:

Remove the pizza from the oven and let it rest for a few minutes before cutting it.

Serve hot and enjoy your dietary and nutritious pizza!

Notes: Lentil flour is rich in protein and fiber, making this pizza a healthy and nutritious choice. Fresh vegetables add essential vitamins and minerals, while the use of light mozzarella or low-fat cheese reduces calorie content without sacrificing taste.

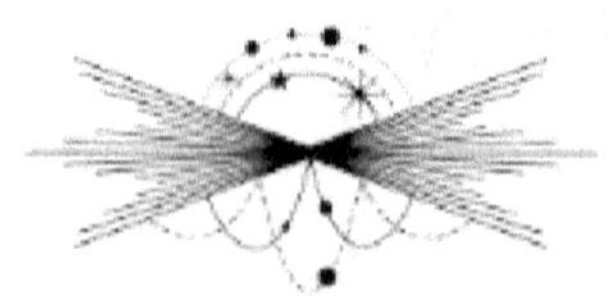

Position yourself in quadrupedal position, with your hands firmly on the ground and your back straight. (Figure 1)

Exhale and do a push-up with your arms, bringing your forehead down to ground and keep your back straight. (Figure 2)

Perform the movement 15 times x 3 times

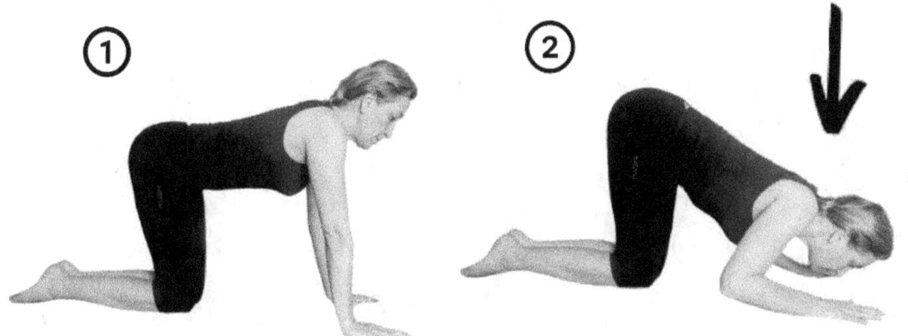

Go to the location of the mountain. (Figure 1)

Exhale and perform a flexion with your arms (Figure 2)

Perform the movement 15 times x 3 times

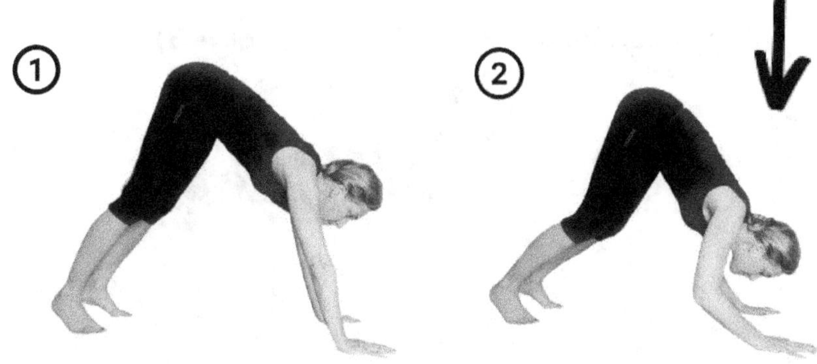

Position yourself in the mid-bridge and listen to the force in your arms and legs. (Figure 1)

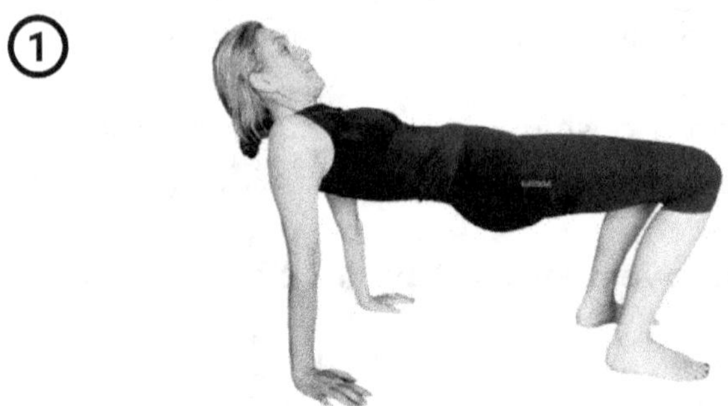

Bend your knees and arms at the same time. Keep your back straight and your gaze forward. (Figure 2)

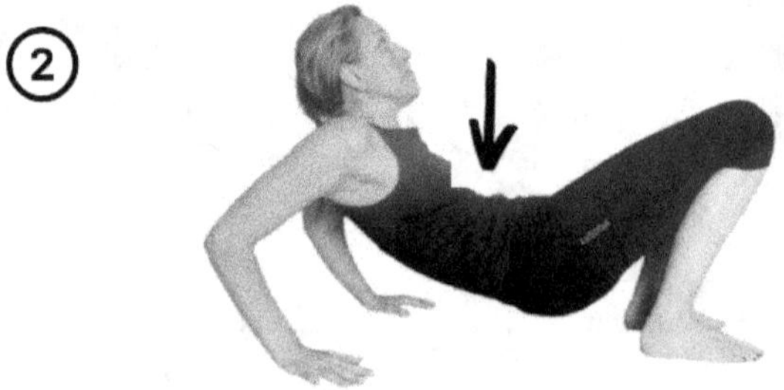

Perform the movement 15 times x 3 times

Exercise 4

Hold this position for a few long breaths (Figure 3)

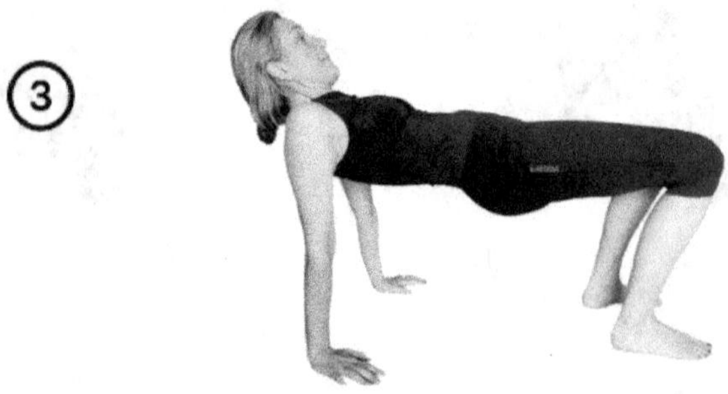

Position yourself in quadrupedal position, with your hands firmly on the ground and your back straight. (Figure 1)

Perform upward lunges with the leg flexed and the toe outstretched. Focus on the radically to the ground as you perform the exercise. Stay balanced and breathe steadily. (Figure 2)

Perform the movement 15 times x 3 times, with the left leg

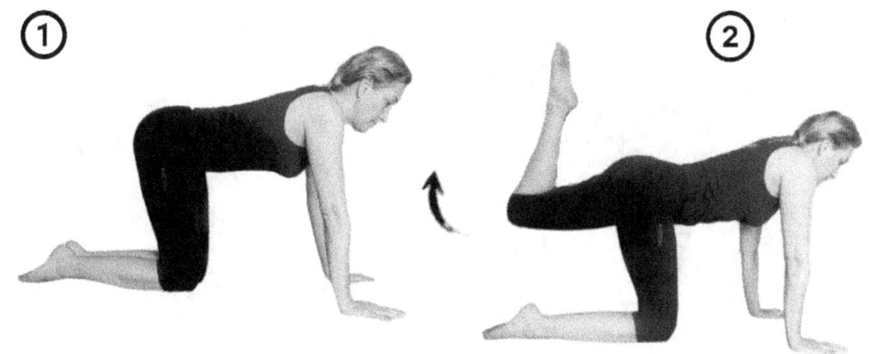

Exercise 6

Perform the movement 15 times x 3 times, with the right leg

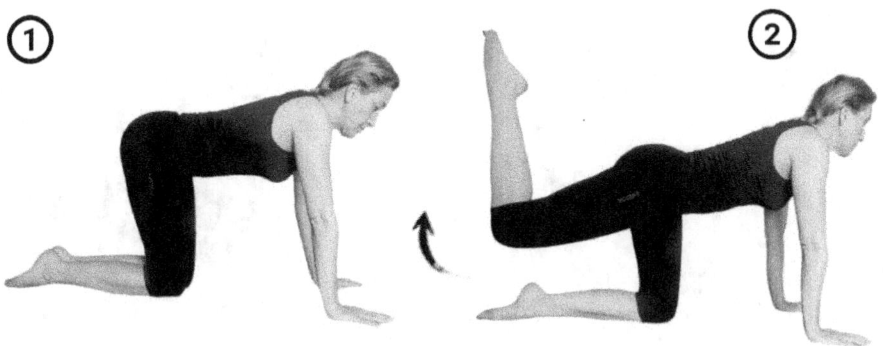

Position yourself in quadrupedal position, with your hands firmly on the ground and your back straight. (Figure 1)

Exhale and bring the knee toward the forehead. The back is curved and the arms are outstretched. Bring attention to the flexibility of the back as it bends and stretches with each movement. (Figure 2)

Perform the movement 15 times x 3 times, with the left leg

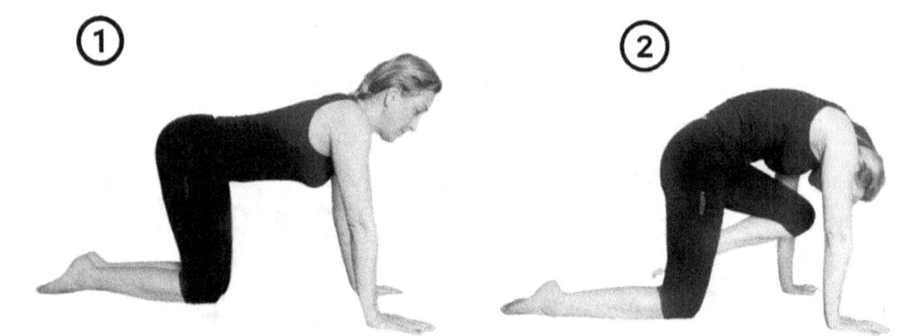

Exercise 8

Perform the movement 15 times x 3 times, with the right leg

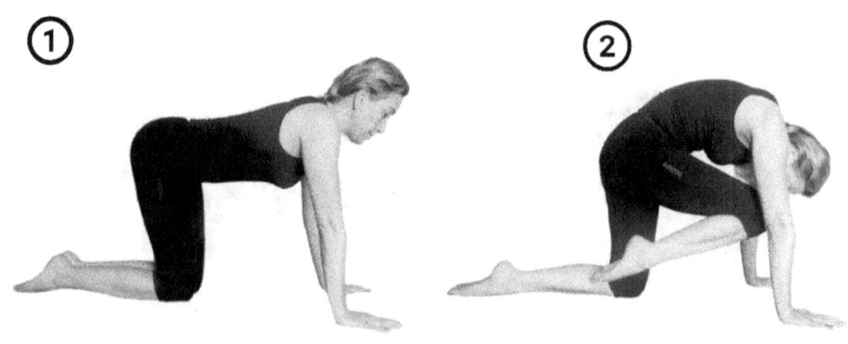

Perform an upward slant with the leg flexed and the toe outstretched (Figure 1)

Then bring the knee toward the forehead. (Figure 2)

Perform the movement 15 times x 3 times, with the left leg

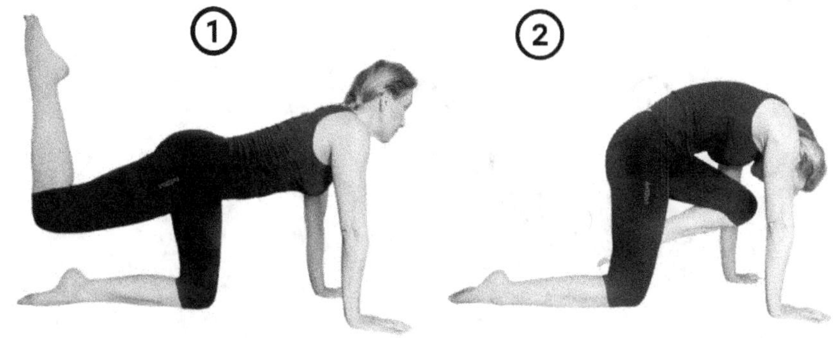

Exercise 10

Perform an upward slant with the leg flexed and the toe outstretched (Figure 1)

Then bring the knee toward the forehead. (Figure 2)

Perform the movement 15 times x 3 times, with the right leg

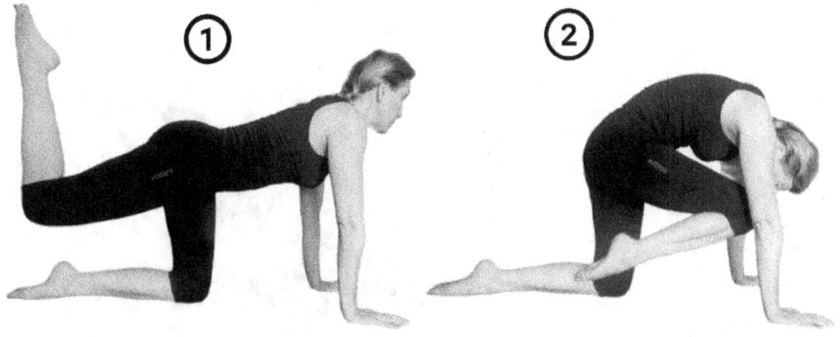

Position yourself sitting on the floor with your back against the floor and your arms along your sides. (Figure 1)

Exhale and lift your shoulders off the floor. Bring your hands past your knees and feel your abdominals contract. (Figure 2)

Perform the movement 15 times x 3 times

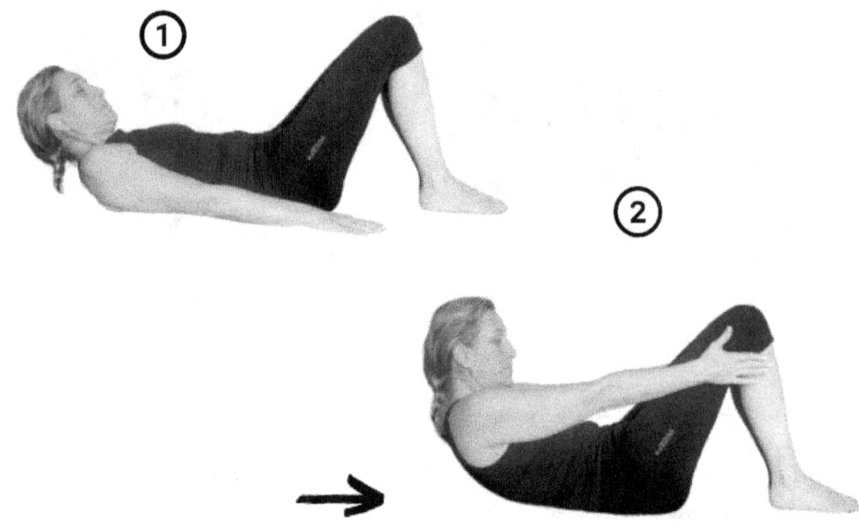

Exercise 12

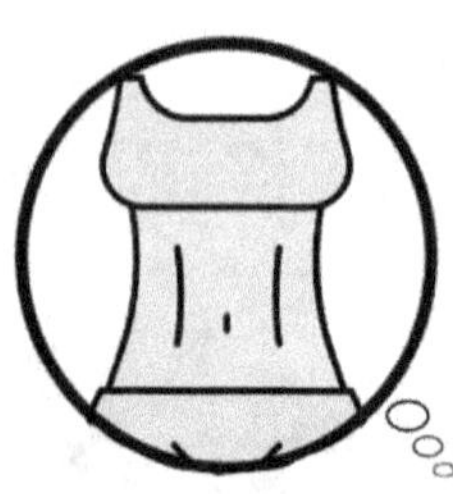

Hold this position for a few long breaths (Figure 3)

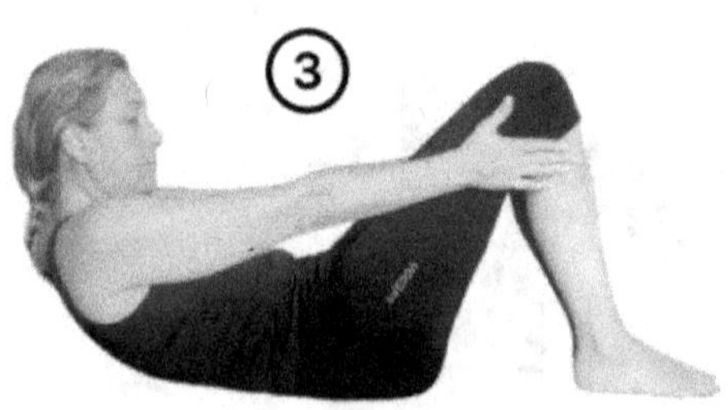

Stand with your back on the floor and legs slightly bent. Keep your eyes closed and visualize your surroundings: the room, walls, furniture and the space around you.

Visualize the surface you are lying on and place your attention on the points of your body that press against that surface. Become aware of each part of your body.

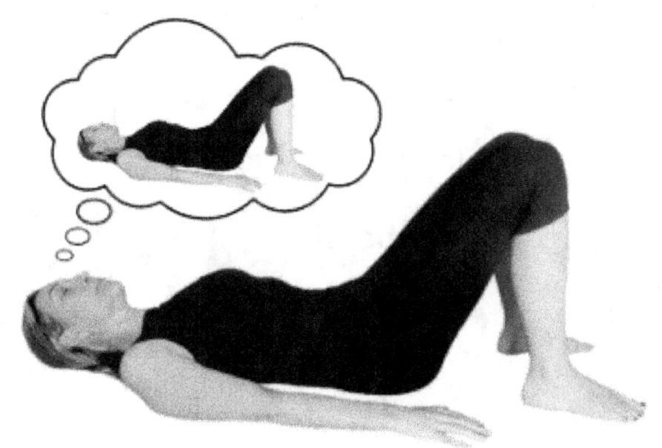

Phrase of the Day

To be repeated several times throughout the day:

"It is never too late to be what you might have been." - George Eliot

Gratification

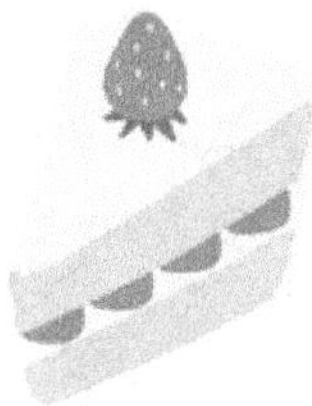

Fancy something sweet? Even on a diet you can have desserts! The important thing is to choose the right one for you. Make a diet cake and eat it in the company of those you love. Stress-free eating is important for your well-being.

Ingredients:

- 300 g of whole wheat flour

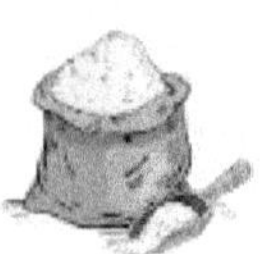

- 200 ml of water

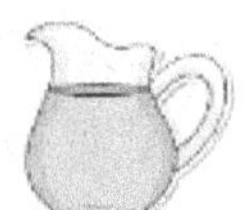

- 100 g of brown sugar (or natural sweetener to taste)

- 50 ml of seed oil

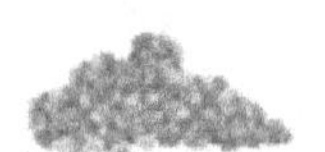

- 1 sachet of baking powder

- Grated zest of 1 lemon (organic)

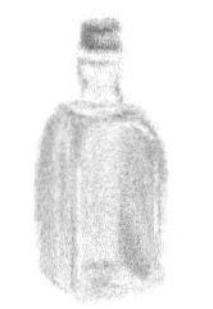

- 1 teaspoon vanilla extract

- A pinch of salt

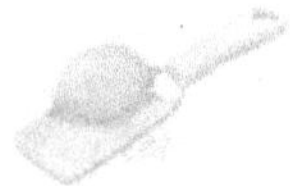

Procedure:

Oven preparation: Preheat the oven to 180°C (350°F). Grease and flour a cake pan about 22-24 cm in diameter.

Dry ingredients: In a large bowl, sift the whole wheat flour and baking powder. Add brown sugar and a pinch of salt, mixing well.

Liquid ingredients: In another bowl, mix the water, seed oil, grated lemon zest and vanilla extract.

Combine the ingredients: Gradually pour the liquid ingredients into the bowl of dry ingredients, stirring with a hand whisk or wooden spoon until smooth and lump-free.

Pour into the cake pan: Transfer the batter into the prepared cake pan, leveling it with a spatula.

Baking: Bake the cake in the preheated oven and bake for about 35 to 40 minutes, or until a toothpick inserted in the center comes out clean.

Cooling: Remove the cake from the oven and let it cool in the cake pan for 10 minutes. Next, transfer it to a wire rack to cool completely.

Suggestions:

Variations: You can enrich the cake with chopped nuts, such as walnuts or almonds, or add dark chocolate chips for an extra touch of flavor.

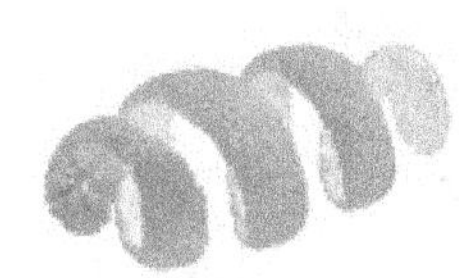

Flavorings: If you prefer, you can replace the lemon zest with orange or add a pinch of cinnamon for a different flavor.

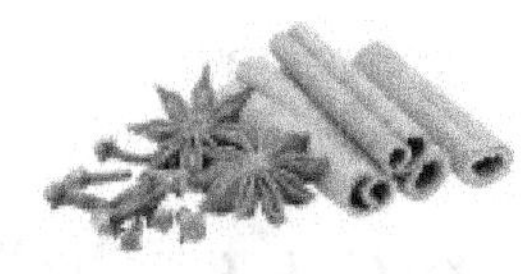

This cake is light, dairy-free and ideal for those who wish to maintain a balanced diet without sacrificing the pleasure of a homemade dessert.

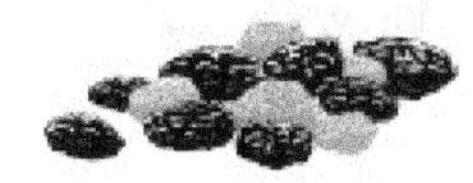

Enjoy your meal!

The Position of the Warrior

The Warrior posture, which you will perform in this somatic practice, also known as "Virabhadrasana" in yoga, is a powerful and dynamic posture that involves the whole body. There are several variations of this posture.

Fat accumulation in the Thighs according to Psychosomatics:

According to psychosomatics, fat accumulation in the thighs may be related to feelings of insecurity and protection. The thighs represent movement and advancement in life, so retaining fat in this area may indicate an unconscious desire for stability and grounding, or resistance to moving forward in life.

Why Practice the Warrior's Posture:

Muscle Stimulation: Tones the thigh muscles, improving their definition.

Improved Circulation: Increases blood flow in the legs, helping to reduce water retention and fat.

Confidence and Inner Strength: Strengthens determination and courage, helping to overcome mental barriers related to insecurity.

Regularly incorporating the Warrior pose into your exercise routine can be an effective way to slim your thighs, increase your physical and mental strength, and address the root causes of fat accumulation in this area.

Exercise 1

Position yourself spread-legged with your hands resting on your knees. Listen to the floor under your feet and keep your back straight. Keep your toes open. (Figure 1)

Exhale and perform a knee bend. Keep your gaze facing forward. Feel your thigh muscles tense and active. (Figure 2)

Perform the movement 15 times x 3 times, with the left leg forward

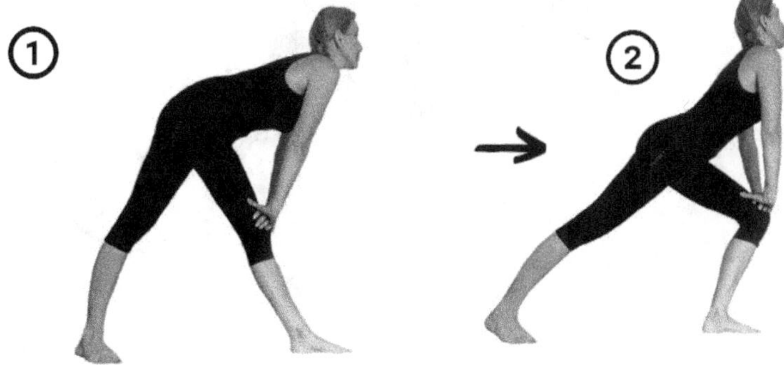

Exercise 2

Perform the movement 15 times x 3 times, with the right leg forward

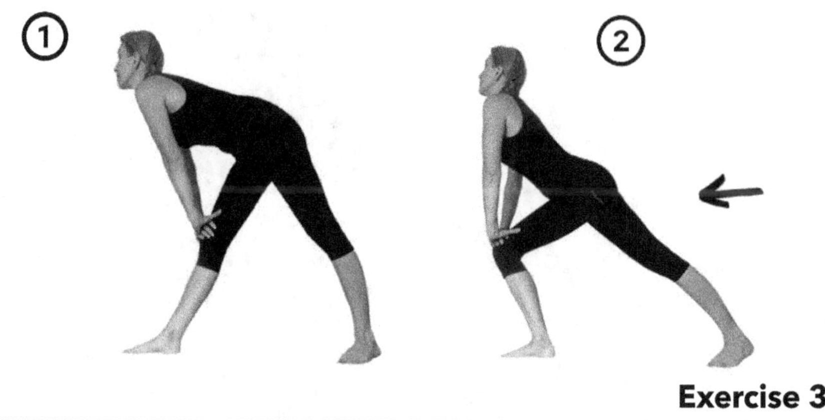

Exercise 3

Hold this position, with the right leg forward, for a few long breaths

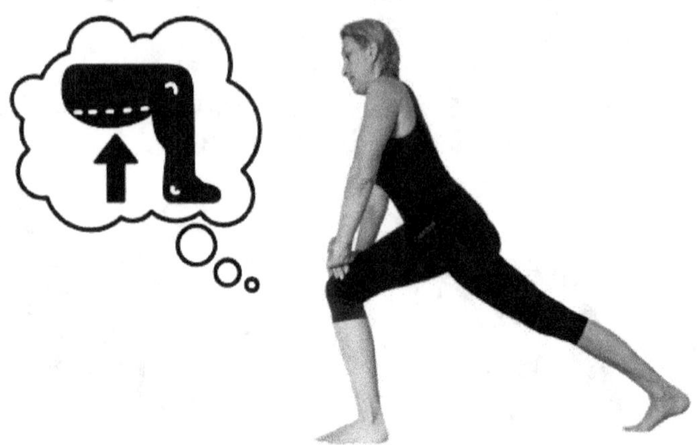

Hold this position, with the left leg forward, for a few long breaths

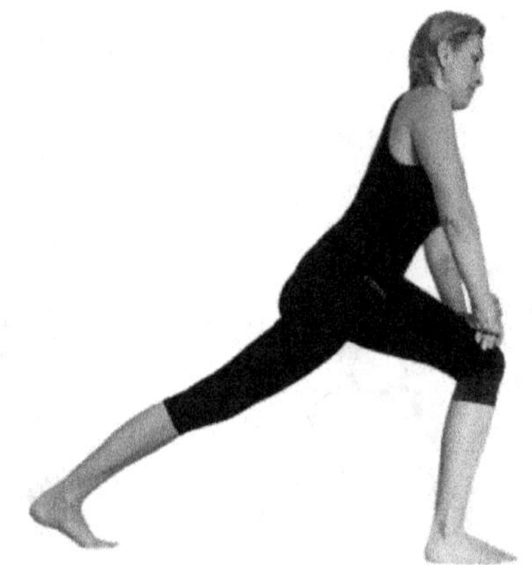

Position yourself with your legs spread apart with your hands resting on the floor. Feel the muscles and tendons in your legs and back stretch. (Figure 1)

Hold this position for a few breaths, with the right leg forward

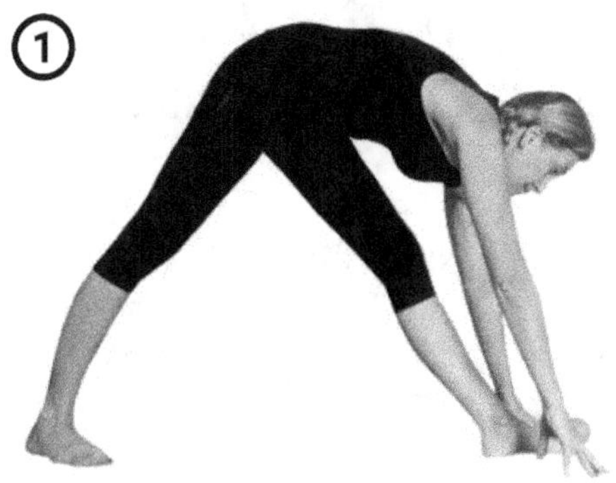

Exercise 6

Hold this position for a few breaths, with the left leg forward

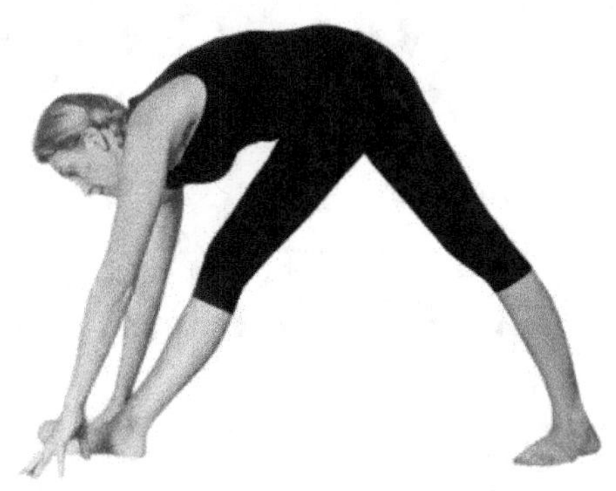

Position yourself with legs spread apart with your hands resting on the ground. (Figure 1)

Exhale and perform knee flexion. (Figure 2)

Perform the movement 15 times x 3 times, with the left leg forward

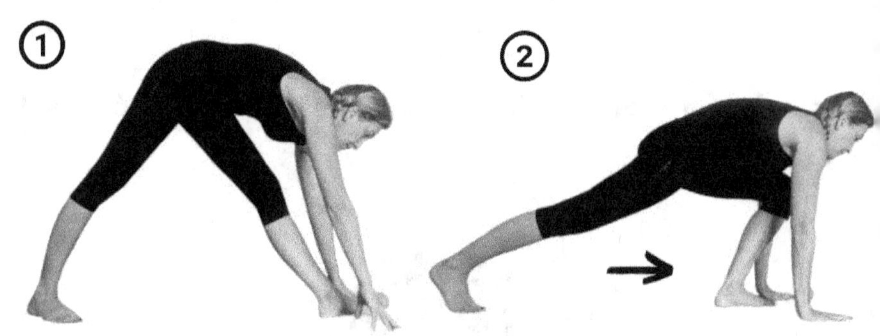

Perform the movement 15 times x 3 times, with the right leg forward

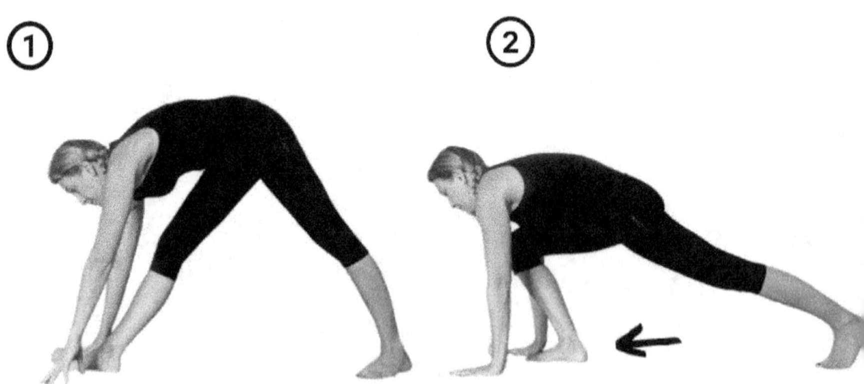

Perform all the previous exercises in sequence, following the slow rhythm of deep breathing.

Perform the movement 15 times x 3 times

Leg forward: right

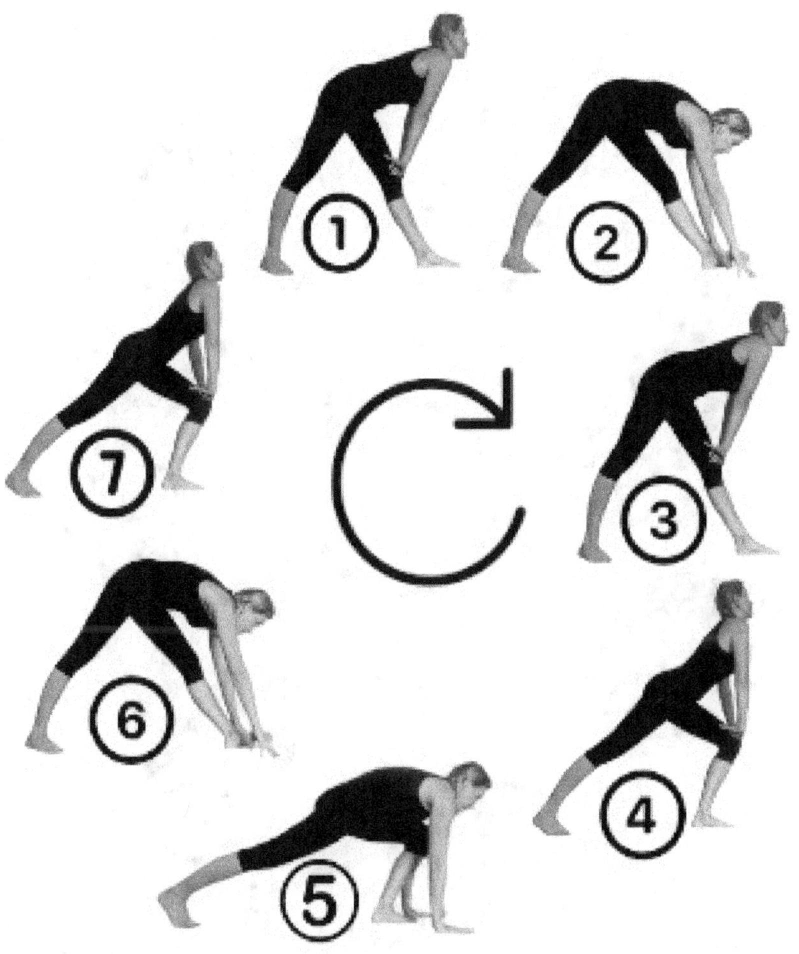

Perform all the previous exercises in sequence, following the slow rhythm of deep breathing.

Perform the movement 15 times x 3 times

Leg forward: left

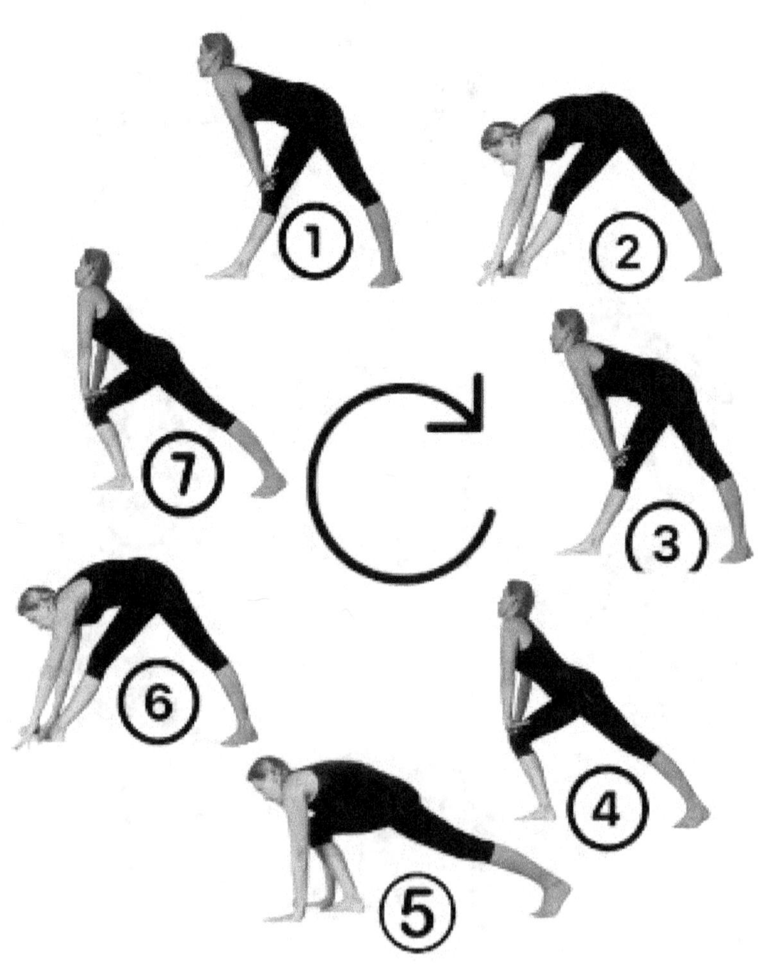

Position yourself with legs apart, knees flexed and elbows resting against knees. Bring your palms together in prayer in front of you. Keep your gaze forward and your back straight. Feel new strength and energy supporting your body.

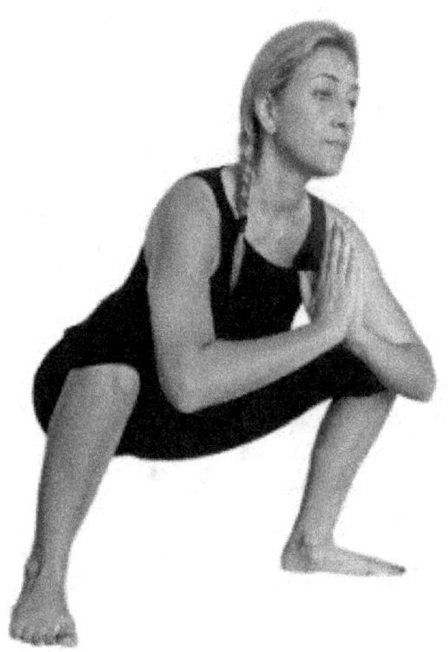

Phrase of the Day

To be repeated several times throughout the day:

"Every morning you have two choices: continue sleeping with your dreams or wake up and chase them." - Anonymous

Gratification

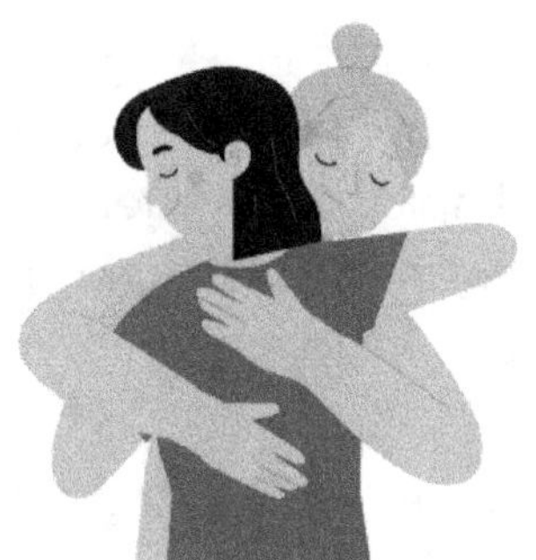

Hug a loved one for at least 30 seconds.

Hugging is an extraordinarily powerful form of human connection. Whether hugging a loved one, a pet, or even an object that evokes fond memories, such as a blanket, pillow, or garment, the power of this simple gesture can have a profound impact on your emotional well-being.

Why Embrace is Helpful

Hugs activate the production of oxytocin, also known as the "love hormone," which promotes feelings of affection, trust and security. This hormone helps reduce levels of cortisol, the stress hormone, thereby promoting a sense of calm and relaxation. In a weight-loss diet context, stress reduction is crucial, as chronic stress can lead to impulsive eating behaviors and increased appetite for unhealthy foods.

Embracing a Loved One

When you hug a loved one, it creates a moment of intimacy and connection that can strengthen your emotional support. This positive interaction not only improves your mood, but can also motivate you to continue your weight loss journey with renewed determination. The physical and emotional closeness experienced during a hug can reduce feelings of loneliness and anxiety often associated with the challenges of lifestyle change.

Hugging a Pet

Pets offer a unique kind of unconditional affection. Hugging your dog or cat can reduce stress and increase your sense of well-being. Animals are nonjudgmental, and their simple, direct affection can provide great comfort in times of trouble. This connection can also encourage you to maintain a positive attitude and stay motivated in your weight loss journey.

Embracing a Blanket, Pillow or Garment

Hugging a blanket, pillow or garment that reminds you of someone you loved very much can also have similar beneficial effects. These objects evoke feelings of safety and comfort, bringing back fond and loving memories. This can help reduce anxiety and create a positive emotional environment that supports your ability to cope with diet and life challenges.

The Importance of Embracing in the Slimming Diet.

Integrating hugs into your daily routine , during a weight-loss diet, can offer you valuable emotional support. Physical contact and emotional connection can relieve stress, improve mood, and increase your psychological resilience. This not only helps you maintain motivation, but also allows you to face the challenges of lifestyle change with greater serenity and determination.

In conclusion, the power of hugging should not be underestimated as it is in modern society, where everyone is in a rush and physical contact is very limited.

Dear readers,

you have come to the end of this journey, a journey that has explored the deepest meanderings of physical and mental well-being. Every page of this book has been written with the intention of providing you with valuable tools and effective practices to improve your life, to embrace health and happiness with a renewed awareness.

You can use this knowledge while performing exercises in the gym, walking or other types of physical exercises.

We also discovered together the power of the mind-body connection, the importance of grounding, and the comfort in a simple hug. We explored relaxation techniques, healthy recipes, and mindfulness practices that can transform your daily life.

The journey to wellness is personal and unique to each of you, but I hope the words shared here have inspired and guided you toward a healthier and happier version of yourself. Every small step, every positive habit you adopt, is a piece that contributes to your mosaic of health and serenity.

Remember, mindfulness and self-love are the pillars of a balanced life. Continue to cultivate these qualities, day after day, and allow yourself to grow and flourish in all your glory.

Thank you for sharing this journey with me. I wish you all the best on your continued journey to wellness and happiness.

With gratitude,

Maia Solara

Maia Solara is an author and somatic healing practitioner dedicated to promoting holistic wellness through body awareness and integrative healing.

With a background in alternative healing, he has explored disciplines such as Ayurveda and Traditional Chinese Medicine, understanding the importance of balance between mind, body and spirit in healing trauma.

Maia has written numerous books and articles on coping with and overcoming trauma through somatic exercises, mindfulness and relaxation practices. Her compassionate and scientific approach has helped many people find inner peace and build more resilient and harmonious lives.

In addition to writing, Maia leads classes, sharing her knowledge and techniques to promote wellness and healing. With a deep dedication to her mission, Maia Solara continues to inspire and guide anyone who wishes to embark on a path of personal growth and transformation.

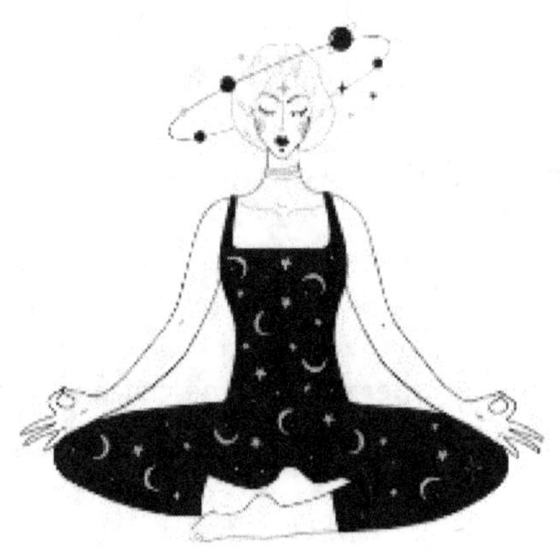

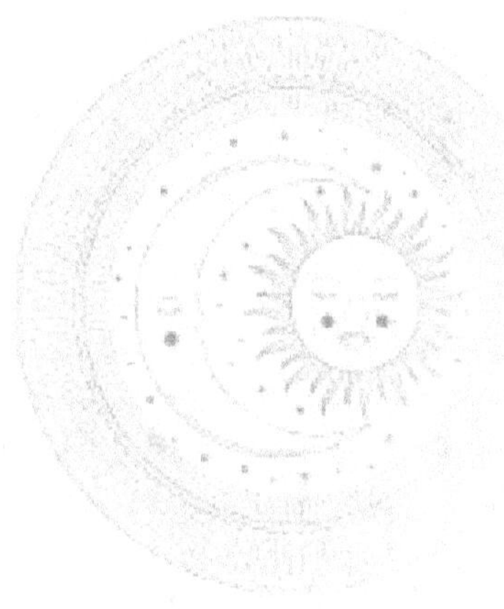